Springer Series on the Teaching of Nursing

Diane O. McGivern, RN, PhD, FAAN, Series Editor
New York University Division of Nursing

Advisory Board: Ellen Baer, PhD, RN, FAAN; Carla Mariano, EdD, RN, AHN-C, FAAIM; Janet A. Rodgers, PhD, RN, FAAN; Alice Adam Young, PhD, RN

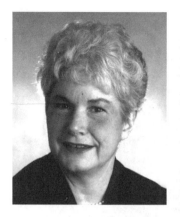

Carol Noll Hoskins, Phd, RN, FAAN, is Professor Emeritus, Division of Nursing, The Steinhardt School of Education at New York University. She is the author of several books, two measures of interactive behaviors in the partner relationship, and numerous articles. Professor Hoskins is principal investigator for a program of breast cancer research. Part I (1990–1994) was used to develop a four-part instructional videotape series, *Journey to Recovery: For Women with Breast Cancer and Their Partners* (1995–1997). The phase-specific content is applicable to the diagnostic, postsurgical, adjuvant therapy, and ongoing recovery periods. As principal investigator, Professor Hoskins, along with her research team, completed a pilot study funded by the National Institute for Nursing Research for a randomized clinical trial to study the effectiveness of standardized education by videotape, telephone counseling, or a combination of the two interventions both for women and their partners over time (1998–2001). She serves as principal investigator for a full confirmatory randomized clinical trial funded by the National Cancer Institute (2002–2006). Her international recognition includes a Fulbright Award at the University of Athens (1995) and a Fulbright Senior Specialists Award in Cyprus (2003).

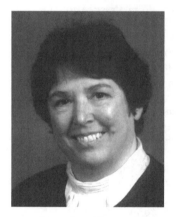

Carla Mariano, EdD, RN, AHN-C, FAAIM, is Associate Professor and Coordinator, Advanced Practice Holistic Nurse Practitioner Program and Scholar in Residence at the John Hartford Institute for Geriatric Nursing, Division of Nursing, The Steinhardt School of Education, New York University. She teaches a doctoral course on Approaches to Qualitative Inquiry; guides numerous doctoral dissertations using qualitative methodology; and teaches master's courses on theoretical foundations of holistic nursing, complementary/alternative modalities, and crisis theory and intervention. Dr. Mariano has conducted qualitative research in the fields of natural healing, gerontology, and interdisciplinarity and has presented her research nationally and internationally. Dr. Mariano has numerous publications, including those on the Qualitative Research Process, The Case Study Method, Instructional Strategies/ Curricular Considerations for Teaching Qualitative Research, Holistic Healing Practices, Holistic Ethics and Research, Interdisciplinary Collaboration, and aging. She was inducted into the Teachers College Columbia University Hall of Fame; is the recipient of the Distinguished Achievement in Nursing Education Award from Teachers College, Columbia University; the Rose and George Doval Award for Excellence in Education; and the 2003–2004 Holistic Nurse of the Year Award from American Holistic Nurses Association.

RESEARCH IN NURSING AND HEALTH

UNDERSTANDING AND USING
QUANTITATIVE AND QUALITATIVE METHODS
2ND EDITION

Carol Noll Hoskins, PhD, RN, FAAN
Carla Mariano, EdD, RN, HNC, FAAIM

with Contributors

Springer Series on the
Teaching of Nursing

Springer Publishing Company, Inc.
536 Broadway
New York, NY 10012-3955

Acquisitions Editor: Ruth Chasek
Production Editor: Pamela Lankas
Cover design by Joanne Honigman

04 05 06 07 08/5 4 3 2 1

Library of Congress Cataloging-in-Publication Data

Research in nursing and health : understanding and using quantitative and qualitative methods / [edited by] Carol Noll Hoskins, Carla Mariano — 2nd ed.
    p. cm. — (Springer series on the teaching of nursing)
    Previous ed. entitled: Developing research in nursing and health.
    Includes bibliographical references and index.
    ISBN 0-8261-1616-7 (alk. paper)
    1. Nursing—Research—Methodology.
    [DNLM: 1. Nursing Research—methods. 2. Research Design. WY 20 5 D4895 2004]
I. Hoskins, Carol Noll, 1932- II. Mariano, Carla. III. Developing research in nursing and health. IV. Springer series on the teaching of nursing (Unnumbered)
RT81.5.D49 2004
610.73'072—dc22   2004013306

Printed in Canada by Capital City Press.

There are few words to express how much I have learned from my doctoral students over many years of teaching. It was a result of their urging that I decided to write this book. It is dedicated to them with a deep sense of gratitude. I also would like to extend my sincere appreciation to both Ursula Springer and her staff, as well as to Carla Mariano, for their encouragement and belief that the book would make a worthy contribution to doctoral education.

—Carol Noll Hoskins

To students, my inspiration.

To J.B.: My wise, gentle guide to understanding and my continual support.

—Carla Mariano

Contents

CONTENTS

Contributors

Barbara Carty, EdD, RN, FAAN, Clinical Associate Professor, has developed and is presently Coordinator of the Nursing Informatics Program in The Division of Nursing, The Steinhardt School of Education, at New York University. Her clinical research has included an informatics model that examines outcomes of care for patients with congestive heart failure, the development of an informatics evaluation tool for data sets for patient care, a national survey of informatics technologies and strategies in graduate and undergraduate programs and student outcomes in the application of distance learning methodologies. Dr. Carty has presented and written on informatics both nationally and internationally. She has authored a book: *Nursing Informatics: Education for Practice*, which received the AJN Book of the Year Award in 2002.

Joseph Giacquinta, EdD, is Professor Emeritus, Department of Educational Sociology, The Steinhardt School of Education at New York University. He has taught graduate courses on both survey research and case study design. Among his publications are *Implementing Organizational Innovations* (1971) and *Beyond Technology's Promise* (1993). He was the recipient of the New York University Professor of the Year Award in 2001.

Susan Kaplan Jacobs, MLS, RN, is the Health Sciences Librarian at the Elmer Holmes Bobst Library, New York University, with responsibility for liaison, collection development, instruction, and reference for the Division of Nursing, Department of Physical Therapy, Department of Occupational Therapy, and Department of Speech-Language Pathology and Audiology at NYU's Steinhardt School of Education. She is a member of the Medical Library Association's NAHRS Task Force to Map the Literature of Nursing, serves as a Medical Library Association representative to the Interagency Council on Information Resources for Nursing (ICIRN), and has collaborated with nursing faculty on presentations and manuscripts.

Preface

Nursing research continues to grow at a remarkable rate. Knowledge and technological advances have exploded, new methods of inquiry have been developed, and research texts have proliferated. This book offers the reader a synopsis of research appreciating both the science and art of inquiry. It includes the research process that builds knowledge through the quantitative method and that which extends humanistic understanding through qualitative investigations. Dr. Carol Noll Hoskins authored those sections on quantitative research. Dr. Carla Mariano authored the qualitative research sections.

The book was designed to present the basic elements of conducting and understanding nursing research using an expeditious and useful reference format. The primary motivation for the book came from many students in the Program in Research and Theory Development in Nursing at New York University, for which Dr. Hoskins served as the Director from 1985 to 1990. The first versions of the chapters emerged from the request of students for seminars in the doctoral program reinforced by written handouts that were succinct and easy to use. Over the years, the guides were revised and edited and used in other countries, including academic settings in Thailand, India, Finland, Greece, and Cyprus. Although it was originally created for doctoral students, the material can be used by students at the baccalaureate and master's levels, and by practicing nurses.

Chapter 1 provides a review of the basic reasons nurses need to be involved as consumers or designers of research. The challenge of constant evaluation of patient care and how it might be revised in the interest of improving outcomes in patients and families is stressed.

In chapter 2, the complexities of identifying and refining a research question are addressed. The research question, whether quantitative or qualitative, provides direction to the entire study, including the design that will be used to seek answers. Although there are various techniques and views on conducting a literature review, progress has been enormous in executing the process. Content on the literature review is presented and discussed in chapter 3. Most investigators agree that the main aim for a review of the literature should be the acquisition of a comprehensive knowledge of the work that has already been completed. Accomplishing this objective will enable an investigator to avoid the risk of developing a study and interpreting the findings in a relative vacuum.

The next two chapters are focused on the methodological aspects of planning and conducting both quantitative and qualitative research. There is a great deal of information about research designs, sampling, measurement, data analysis and interpretations. The main points are outlined and intended to serve as a starting point, while those who seek more information can consult more comprehensive and specialized references. In the recent past, the amount to be learned about the methodological aspects of research, particularly in terms of design and analyses of data, has been massive. The focus on psychometrics and development of measures appropriate for assessing predictors and outcomes of interest to nursing has grown exponentially. There is an increasing need to set standards for developing and evaluating instruments for validity, reliability, and sound theoretical foundations. And yet many phenomena of concern to nursing remain unexplored and/or undocumented, necessitating the use of increasingly evolving and complex qualitative methods for expanding the discipline's developing body of knowledge. The increased emphasis on the ethics involved in conducting human research also is addressed. With increased governmental monitoring of the ethics of research and the emphasis on privacy issues all investigators are required to pay particular attention to these aspects of the research process.

Finally, the content in specific chapters is supplemented by two chapters in which guidelines for critiquing studies with actual exemplar studies are presented. Criteria for rigor of both qualitative and quantitative research are identified; however, not all research meets the standards that have been set for methodological and theoretical rigor, regardless of the discipline. Therefore the responsibility rests with the practitioner for application of high standards prior to implementing the results of a study.

Those who read this book will be the researchers and educators of research in the future. As there are no single answers to our comprehensive questions in nursing, there are no single methods for answering those questions. It is the hope of the authors that this book may provide a helpful guide in your research endeavors.

CAROL NOLL HOSKINS AND CARLA MARIANO

1
Introduction to Research

Increasingly, the research process has been conducted under enormous pressures of time, competition for funds, and other factors that have had a tremendous influence on society in general. Computer technology and databases are intended to make previous studies, including theoretical framework, design, measurement, sample, analyses, and findings, available in the aggregate within moments. Secondary reviews of literature are available for those who decide against primary sources. Although theory development remains an important part of the development and conduct of research, thoughtful attention to the process, as well as other components of the process, becomes more and more problematic.

In Chapter 1, the basic reasons for conducting nursing research are reviewed. Although they are not new, they remain sound. Of increasing importance is research on outcomes that are sensitive measures of nursing practice. Further, in the world of managed care, health care system variables as antecedents to outcomes demand increasing attention in nursing research.

In keeping with the pace of modern times, the chapters in this book are primarily in outline form. The reader can, with ease, note the essential points for each topic without the distraction of lengthy text. The reader is strongly urged, however, to seek other references when further information is required. A list of some basic texts is provided in the References.

I. INTRODUCTION TO RESEARCH IN NURSING

    A.   Importance of research to nursing

        1.   Practice

            a.   Understand clients' experiences
            b.   Quality of care and outcomes
            c.   Cost effectiveness of care

        2.   Professionalism

            a.   Scientific base for practice
            b.   Body of knowledge that is distinct from other professions

3.   Accountability

    a.   Base decisions and actions in practice, administration, and education on scientifically documented knowledge
    b.   Seek scientific answers to professional issues
    c.   Read the scientific literature for new knowledge and apply to nursing practice, administration, and education

4.   Social relevance of nursing

    a.   Nursing, more than ever, is required by consumers and sources of reimbursement to document its role in the delivery of health services

        —   Of what benefit is nursing?
        —   Can it be documented that nursing care makes a difference?
        —   Of what social and practical relevance is nursing?

In summary, most nurses in the United States agree that a large component of nursing practice is—or should be—based on science and that scientific knowledge is developed through research. The research process is a method for posing scientific questions and seeking answers to them. It is a critical function for any profession that claims to base its practice on science.

Without research programs to build its knowledge, a profession is limited to existing knowledge that is often inadequate, or to knowledge developed by other disciplines that may not be appropriate to the problems of the professional practice in question.

B.   Kinds of research

1.   Basic

    a.   Establish new knowledge or facts
    b.   Develop theories or conceptual frameworks
    c.   Results are not immediately applicable to real-world situations

2.   Applied

    a.   Attempts to find solutions to practical problems
    b.   Applies new knowledge relatively soon

II.   RELATIONSHIP OF THEORY TO QUANTITATIVE RESEARCH

The theoretical framework within which a given problem is lodged is of crucial importance in every stage of the research. A theory is a systematic explanation of some phenomenon, broader and more complex than a fact. It identifies the variables needed to explain the phenomenon of interest and suggests the nature of the relationships among the variables.

"If a particular problem on which one proposes to do research is not related to an existing theory, does not grow out of an existing theory, is not contained within a newly formed theory, or does not appear capable of altering or confirming a theory, it is most likely irrelevant, useless, and unimportant for consideration as a research problem, especially if an experimental or explanatory nature" (Geitgey & Metz, 1973, pp. 1–5).

A. Theory

    1. Consists of

        a. The interrelationships of what is known to be true from research evidence
        b. What is assumed to be true on the basis of writings by scientists and theoreticians

    2. Serves to

        a. Explain
        b. Predict
        c. Give direction to research by specifying the variables that need to be measured prior to conducting the research
        d. Provide a framework of variables within which the findings may be compared and integrated with the results of other research

    3. Assists in selecting the most appropriate variables from which to design the research and guides in their definition
    4. Determines the statement and direction of the hypotheses and the subsequent interpretation of findings
    5. Provides the theoretical basis for linking variables

        a. The variables may not be arbitrarily linked. They must have empirical or theoretical support for coexistence and testing.
        b. Logic is used in defining the relationships between variables, e.g., if *A is related to B*, and *B is related to C*, then perhaps *A is related to C.*

III. THE NATURE OF QUALITATIVE RESEARCH

A. Characteristics

"The qualitative approach is interactive; context dependent; holistic; flexible, dynamic, and evolving; naturalistic; process oriented; primarily inductive; and descriptive. It has as its foci, perspectives, meanings, uniqueness, and subjective live experiences. Its aim is understanding" (Mariano, 1990, p. 354). Qualitative research methods enable us to explore concepts that we experience in our everyday lives, such as empathy, hope, suffering, caring, fear; to explore these concepts as they are perceived and defined by real people; and to allow people to speak for themselves, thereby emphasizing the human capacity to know (Mariano, 1995).

1. Use of the natural setting
2. Emphasis on exploration and discovery versus testing and verifying predetermined hypotheses
3. Focus on the complexity and wholeness of the phenomenon of human experience—appreciates multiple realities
4. There is an humanistic orientation
5. There is direct, close, and prolonged contact with the participants
6. Attends to temporal, social, and historical contexts
7. The researcher is the human instrument
8. The design emerges
9. Participant observation and in-depth interviewing are frequently used
10. The study generates an understanding of the human experience often through extensive description or grounded theory

2

The Research Question

The most important initial step in developing research is the identification and phrasing of the research question. This is a process that occurs over time as one reviews the literature and examines studies for questions that have been studied previously. Identifying the constructs, understanding how they have been conceptualized, and evaluating the rationale for linking them are key parts of the endeavor. As studies are located and critiqued, the investigators' phrasing of their own research question is likely to be revised a number of times. If there is little or no work on a particular topic of interest, then the investigator needs to consider approaching the research question from a qualitative perspective.

In chapter 2, the sources and characteristics of quantitative and qualitative research questions are presented. Guides are provided for phrasing each kind of question. In the case of a quantitative question, the kinds of hypotheses and criteria for phrasing them are considered. While the outline format is intended to highlight the key points in a succinct manner, the reader needs to remember that the process requires substantial time, care, and thought which, in the long run, will be worth it.

I. SOURCES OF RESEARCH QUESTIONS

    A. Practice
    B. Nursing theory
    C. Literature
    D. Previous research
    E. Nursing models
    F. Phenomena inherent in the human condition
    G. Social concerns

II. THE RESEARCH PROBLEM (QUANTITATIVE)

    A. Consists of *variables* that are

        1. Constructs or properties that are studied in research
        2. A property that takes on different values (varies)

            a. Continuous
            b. Dichotomous

3.   Usually represented by a symbol
4.   Two major kinds

   a.   Independent variable
      — presumed "cause" of the dependent variable
      — referred to as "X"
      — in experimental research, the variable that is manipulated by the experimenter
      — the variable predicted from

   b.   Dependent variable

      — presumed effect of independent variable
      — referred to as "Y"
      — the variable predicted to

III.   THE RESEARCH PROBLEM (QUALITATIVE)

Because the specific problem that actually becomes the focus of the study often *emerges during* the fieldwork, it is likely to be more tentative than in quantitative research.

A.   Aim of the study (qualitative)

   1.   Consists of:

      a.   Description of the focus of inquiry—what is the phenomenon of interest, what is the event or situation or question to be explored?
      b.   Context of the phenomenon—the milieu of the phenomenon
      c.   Context of the researcher

         — researcher's experiences, background, assumptions, preconceptions, intuitions, root of interest in the phenomenon
         — researcher's expertise in the method (including preliminary fieldwork)

      d.   Purpose of the inquiry, e.g., theory building, descriptive base for practice
      e.   Succinct overview of the method selected and rationale for why that method is appropriate for this study
      f.   Significance of inquiring about this phenomenon

         — why is it important to study
         — relevance of the inquiry
         — why is it necessary to utilize a qualitative design

    — contribution of the study to understanding, knowledge, practice, and importance to nursing

    — contribution to knowledge, practice, and policy in this area

IV. PHRASING THE RESEARCH QUESTION (QUANTITATIVE)

A. An interrogative sentence or statement that asks, "What relation exists between two or more variables?"

    Ex. Is social support related to patients' and husbands' psychosocial adjustment to breast cancer?

B. Criteria for research questions

    1. Express a relation between two or more variables
    2. State clearly and unambiguously in question form
    3. Imply possibilities for empirical testing
    4. Specify the nature of the population being studied
    5. Be introduced early in a research report, with a brief statement of the experiential and scientific background that led to the study

V. PHRASING THE RESEARCH QUESTION (QUALITATIVE)

A. Asking the question

A question that asks how an individual or group experiences or perceives a particular phenomenon or creates meaning—what is being experienced, how is it being experienced, how is reality being constructed. Subquestions or areas for exploration may be included.

B. Criteria for research questions

    1. Open-ended or "open-beginning"
    2. Broad
    3. Conducive to context
    4. Oriented to people and the human condition

C. Stating the research question (examples)

    1. What is the nature of . . . ?
    2. What is the description of . . . ?
    3. How do people perceive or experience . . . ?
    4. What is happening here?

VI. HYPOTHESES (QUANTITATIVE)

A. Consists of a conjectural statement of at least one specific relationship between two variables, which can be clearly supported or not supported

B. Criteria for hypotheses

    1. Delineates a relationship between variables
       — the relationship must be empirically testable through collection of data

    2. Conditions implicit in the criteria

       — only one relationship may be specified in a single hypothesis
       — the hypothesis must be written before the study is conducted
       — only words describing an empirically testable relationship may be used in an hypothesis

       Ex. Social support will be positively related to patients' psychosocial adjustment to breast cancer

C. Kinds of hypotheses

    1. Null hypothesis

       a. A statement of no relationship
       b. Denoted as H_0
       c. If a relationship is found, then H_0 is probably false

    2. Research hypothesis (directional)

       a. States the direction that a relationship between two variables is likely to take, meaning that an increase (or decrease) in the independent variable will be related to an increase (or decrease) in the dependent variable
       b. Used when the investigator is interested only in a relationship manifesting itself in one direction and is willing to "throw away" the results in the other direction, no matter how impressive
       c. Has some theoretical or empirical rationale for specifying the direction
       d. Specifies the direction before collecting the data
       e. Gives direction to the design

       Ex. An increase in deep breathing (X_1) and coughing (X_2) will be related to a decreased need for analgesia (Y_1) and length of hospitalization (Y_2) under the condition of preoperative structured teaching as compared to unstructured teaching.

3.   Research hypothesis (nondirectional)

    a.   States that a relationship exists without indicating directionality
    b.   Often used when there is insufficient empirical evidence in support of a directional hypothesis

        Ex.   Patients receiving preoperative instructions differ significantly from patients not receiving preoperative instructions with respect to number of postoperative medication requests.

VII. HYPOTHESES (QUALITATIVE)

A.   Hypotheses may emerge or the researcher may develop hypotheses based on the findings of the study.
B.   In the Grounded Theory method hypotheses are stated to link/relate two or more concepts explaining the what, why, where, and how of a phenomenon. These hypotheses, which are abstractions, are derived from the data and must be validated and further elaborated through continued comparisons of data.

3

A Review of the Literature: Using Online and Print Sources

With the availability of multiple and large electronic databases and knowledge sources, the exercise of performing a literature search has become both more complex and more powerful to the researcher and the end user of the research data, knowledge, and evidence. Whether the researcher is accessing data and knowledge sources to inform a research question, support clinical practice, or develop a research project, more sophisticated skills in information management and literacy are required than in the past. The world of literature and its review have expanded to include varied and numerous digital resources and software tools. These developments enable the researcher to access expert information and knowledge sources.

Chapter 3 will review access to and availability of large data sets and knowledge sources, strategies for locating electronic resources, a definition of research terms, and the development of a theoretical framework based on the knowledge sources.

I. THE LITERATURE REVIEW (QUANTITATIVE)

    A. Primary purposes

        1. Orientation to what is known

            a. Includes identification of assumptions about certain aspects of the phenomenon being studied
            b. Identifies methodologies (research approaches) (e.g., *how* the information, or findings, were found, both qualitative and quantitative)

        2. Provision of a conceptual or theoretical framework

            a. Identify broad conceptual issues related to theoretical frameworks for a specific problem

      3.   Indication of a research approach

          a.   Research design
          b.   Measurement instruments
          c.   Statistical analyses

  B.   Common errors in conducting a literature search that may have implications for the resulting design

      1.   Conducting too cursory a review that overlooks previous studies containing ideas that might improve the proposed research design
      2.   Focusing only on research findings when reading research reports, thus missing valuable information on methods and measures

II.   THE LITERATURE REVIEW (QUALITATIVE)

  A.   Although there are controversial views on conducting a literature review prior to data collection, a preliminary review of the literature for the proposal is useful for a variety of reasons.

      1.   Opens the researcher to the complexity of the phenomenon under investigation
      2.   Introduces the investigator to the context of the phenomenon and the culture of the participants
      3.   Provides additional justification and credence for the study (e.g., illustrates that this particular phenomenon has not been studied before or studied in this manner)
      4.   Signifies how this research will add to the existing knowledge

  B.   It is important that the researcher remain open to the many new ideas, hunches, and emerging concepts that may occur during the actual course of the study.
  C.   In the dissertation, the literature review is far more developed as the findings are compared and contrasted with existing literature and theory.

III. LARGE DATA SETS AND KNOWLEDGE SOURCES

Computer and information technology have made available to the researcher and the clinician a vast world of scientific evidence and knowledge sources that provide the basis of formulating a research question and evidence for clinical practice. The spectrum of evidence can span information from aggregate clinical data repositories to scientific evidence from randomized clinical trials, and sources can range from the individual client experience to aggregate clinical data. In addition, the ability to capture large data sets and apply sophisticated statistical models, as is done in data mining, has resulted in the development of a technique referred to as KDD (Knowledge Discovery through large Data Sets). These techniques will provide researchers with important research data from large clinical repositories as well as national and international data sets (Abbott, 2000; Delaney et al., 2000; Goodwin et al., 2000). An example of this capability is the ANA National Nursing Quality Indicators (NNQI) project.

In researching the literature and evidence, it is a combination of the research method (qualitative or quantitative) and application of the researchers' knowledge and skills that limit or expand the available evidence. For the most part, this chapter will refer to evidence or literature in electronic or digital format, but will also list print sources. Today, by far the majority of sources are digital.

IV.   DIGITAL SOURCES

Digital sources of evidence and research can be classified as

A.   **Bibliographic:** Bibliographic sources consist of print indexes and electronic data-bases (CINAHL, MEDLINE, etc.), structured reports such as trial banks, and synthesized evidence, which includes electronic textbooks and systematic reviews (Cochrane Collaboration, 2003, Joanna Briggs Institute).

B.   **Practice parameters:** Examples of practice parameters include standards of care, practice guidelines, and disease management programs.

C.   **Comparative databases:** Some comparative databases include the National Nursing Quality Indicators Database, Health Plan Employer Data and International Set (HEDIS), and various state and federal planning and health databases (Bakken, 2001).

D.   **Knowledge bases:** Knowledge bases that provide a sophisticated synthesis and mapping of information and knowledge include the genomic knowledge sources (Genbank, Molecular Modeling Database) and to date the only nursing knowledge database, the On-line Journal of Knowledge Synthesis housed at the Virginia Henderson Electronic International Nursing Library of Sigma Theta Tau. A listing of these electronic and print sources is found in Table 3.1.

V.   KEY SOURCES AND STRATEGIES FOR LOCATING NURSING AND RELATED LITERATURE

When conducting a search in the literature of nursing research, one must keep in mind the interdisciplinary nature of nursing practice. Nursing research is published in nursing journals as well as in multidisciplinary publications; research relevant to nursing practice is also published by non-nurses. Thus, a review of the literature should include consideration of the bibliographic databases for nursing and biomedicine, as well as the social sciences and humanities. The journal literature is best accessed via electronic databases, whereas other primary sources may be located by searching research library catalogs. A semiannual list of "Essential Nursing References" will lead the researcher to core works for background information to supplement a current literature search (Allen et al., 2002).

TABLE 3.1 Electronic and Print Resources

Resource/Publisher	URL	Description
Allied and Complementary Medicine Database (AMED) London: Health Care Information Service of the British Library. • Selective years covered for individual disciplines back to 1985. • Access by subscription.	*http://www.bl.uk/ services/information/ amed.html*	References to articles in more than 500 journals, many not indexed by other biomedical sources. Mainly European focus with the majority of titles in English, for the areas of complementary medicine, physical therapy, occupational therapy, rehabilitation, podiatry, palliative care, speech and language therapy. Indexing terms based on Medline MESH vocabulary.
BNIplus (British Nursing Index) Dorset: BNI Publications. • Updated: monthly. • Years covered: 1987–present. • Access by subscription.	*http://www.bniplus. co.uk/index.html*	Covers British publications and other English language titles from over 220 British nursing and midwifery titles along with major English language journals. Includes articles relevant to nurses and midwives from medical journals and those for healthcare management and professions allied to medicine.
Centers for Disease Control and Prevention • Free Web site.	*http://www.cdc.gov/*	As "the lead federal agency for protecting the health and safety of people—at home and abroad," the CDC site gives credible information to link users to disease, travel, and emergency information, health topics A to Z, and links to the full text of *Morbidity and Mortality Weekly Report (MMWR)*.
CINAHL® Glendale, CA; Cinahl Information Systems • Years covered: 1982–present. • Updated: weekly. Print counterpart: *Cumulative Index to Nursing and Allied Health Literature,* 1956–present. • Access via individual or institutional subscription.	*http://www.cinahl.com/*	Citations for the subjects of nursing, allied health, biomedicine, alternative/complementary medicine, consumer health and health sciences librarianship. Coverage of more than 2400 journals (more than 1600 current journals), as well as selected original and full-text material such as selected state nursing journals, newsletters, standards of practice, practice acts, government publications, research instruments and patient education material.

(continued)

TABLE 3.1 *(continued)*

Resource/Publisher	URL	Description
Cochrane Library Oxford, U.K.: The Cochrane Collaboration. • Updated quarterly. Each issue of the Cochrane Database of Systematic Reviews contains new and updated reviews and protocols. As new evidence becomes available, individual reviews are updated. • Abstracts freely available at *http:// www.cochrane.org/* • Full reviews available via subscription.	*http:// www.cochrane.org*	Includes a collection of regularly updated databases of evidence-based information including the full text of the Cochrane Database of Systematic Reviews. The reviews are presented as complete reviews regularly prepared, updated and updated by Collaborative Review Groups, and protocols for reviews currently being prepared (all include an expected date of completion). Protocols are the background, objectives and methods of reviews in preparation.
Dissertation Abstracts International Ann Arbor, MI: UMI® • Years covered: 1861–present. • Updated: monthly. • Access by subscription.	*http://www.umi.com/*	Abstracts of doctoral dissertations accepted by American universities. Includes master's theses from 1988 forward. Over 47,000 dissertations and 12,000 theses added annually.
Embase Elsevier Science B.V. • Years covered: 1980–present. • Updated: weekly. • Print counterpart *Excerpta Medica* abstract journals, some covered back to 1947 • Access by subscription.	*http://www.embase.com*	Embase, the electronic version of the *Excerpta Medica,* indexes over 3500 international journals in the following fields: drug research, pharmacology, pharmaceutics, toxicology, clinical and experimental human medicine, health policy and management, public health, occupational health, environmental health, drug dependence and abuse, psychiatry, forensic medicine, and biomedical engineering/instrumentation. Selective coverage for nursing, dentistry, veterinary medicine, psychology, and alternative medicine. Nursing researchers attempting to uncover everything about a topic should include an Embase search as part of their literature review.

TABLE 3.1 *(continued)*

Resource/Publisher	URL	Description
ERIC U.S. Department of Education, Rockville, MD • Electronically accessible from 1966–present. Print counterparts: *Current Index to Journals in Education (CIJE),* 1969 to present (for journal articles); *Resources in Education (RIE),* 1966 to present (for research reports). • Available free on the internet and via commercial vendors.	*http://www.eric.ed.gov/*	Bibliographic database of more than 1 million abstracts of education-related documents and journal articles, as well as unpublished reports, available in print or microfiche. Of interest to nurses are materials on the disabled, nursing education, and early childhood.
Essential Nursing References • Free Web site.	*http://www.nln.org/ nlnjournal/ nursingreferences.htm*	Biennial list of core references (both print and electronic) to support nursing research, education, administration, and practice, published by the Interagency Council on Information Resources for Nursing.
Grey Literature Page • Free Web Site.	*http://www.nyam.org/ library/greyreport.shtml*	Links to the Grey Literature Report, a quarterly guide to grey or "fugitive" literature published by organizations and agencies in the fields of Health Policy and Public Health. Links to information such as preprints and statistical reports not published or conventionally indexed by commercial publishers.
Health and Psychosocial Instruments (HAPI). Pittsburgh, PA: Behavioral Measurement Database Services. • Years covered: 1985–present, with many earlier measures. • Updated: quarterly. • Access by subscription.	Email: *bmdshapi@aol. com*	Indexes measurement instruments (i.e., questionnaires, interview schedules, checklists, index measures, coding schemes/manuals, rating scales, projective techniques, vignettes/scenarios, tests) in the health fields, psychosocial sciences, organizational behavior, and library and information science.

(continued)

TABLE 3.1 *(continued)*

Resource/Publisher	URL	Description
Health on the Net Foundation • Free Web site.	*http://www.hon.ch/*	A portal for reliable healthcare information, its HON Code of Conduct provides a multilingual set of principles to "hold Web site developers to basic ethical standards in the presentation of information," and to "help make sure readers always know the source and the purpose of the data they are reading."
Health Plan Employer Data and International Set (HEDIS)	*http://www.ncqa.org/ Programs/HEDIS/*	Sponsored by the National Committee for Quality Assurance (NCQA). A set of standardized performance measures and data that compares the performance of managed health care organizations. It provides purchasers and consumers with information to compare and evaluate the performance of managed health care plans.
HealthSTAR Ovid Sandy, UT: Ovid Technologies, Inc. • Years covered: 1975–present. • Print counterpart: *Hospital Literature Index* 1957–2000, Chicago, IL: American Hospital Association. • Access by subscription. Years 2000–present freely accessible via NLM's PubMed	*http://www.ovid.com http://pubmed.gov/.*	Bibliographic database of published literature on health services, technology, administration, and research, Ovid Healthstar continues the National Library of Medicine's (NLM) now-defunct HealthSTAR database. It focuses on both the clinical and non-clinical aspects of health care delivery. HealthSTAR (Health Services Technology, Administration, and Research) was a bibliographic database that resided separately available from the National Library of Medicine from February 1994 (originally called HSTAR) to December 2000. Materials that comprised HealthSTAR have now migrated to other National Library of Medicine online sources. Journal citations for health services, technology, administration, and research are added weekly to NLM's PubMed (*http://pubmed.gov/*)
Interagency Collaborative on Nursing Statistics (ICONS) • Free Web site.	*http:// www.iconsdata.org/*	An association of individuals from a variety of organizations promotes the generation and utilization of data, information, and research about nurses, nursing education, and the nursing workforce.

TABLE 3.1 *(continued)*

Resource/Publisher	URL	Description
Joanna Briggs Institute • Free Web site.	*http://www.joannabriggs.edu.au/about/coll_centres.php*	An international collaboration of evidence libraries that support evidence-based and best practice. The database includes systematic reviews as well as promoting primary research.
MEDLINE (1966–present). Bethesda, MD: U.S. National Library of Medicine. • Free internet access; also available via commercial interfaces. • Updated: weekly. Pre-1966 citations are found in the print *Index Medicus*	*http://www.pubmed.gov*	The premier biomedical database includes over 11 million citations covering the fields of medicine, nursing, dentistry, veterinary medicine, the health care system, and the preclinical sciences. MEDLINE contains bibliographic citations and author abstracts from more than 4,600 biomedical journals published in the United States and 70 other countries. Includes records from the now ceased *International Nursing Index* (1966–2000). Citations from the pre-1966 literature continue to be added to Medline.
Medlineplus Bethesda, MD: U.S. National Library of Medicine and the National Institutes of Health. • Free Web site.	*http://medlineplus.gov/*	Oriented toward the information needs of consumers and produced by the National Library of Medicine and the National Institutes of Health, links to patient information, interactive health tutorials and support groups on over 600 diseases and conditions, including Spanish language information, a directory of prescription and nonprescription drugs (from the USP DI®). Advice for the Patient®, a product of the United States Pharmacopeia (USP), health information from the media, and links to thousands of clinical trials. A good resource for patients' information.
Medscape-Nursing • Free Web Site; free registration required for some features.	*http://www.medscape.com/nurseshome*	Specialty home page with article summaries, news alerts, a library of abstracts and selected articles from nursing journals, links to nursing conference information, continuing education, and resources for advanced practice nurses.

(continued)

TABLE 3.1   *(continued)*

Resource/Publisher	URL	Description
Mental Measurements Yearbook (MMY) Lincoln, NE: Buros Institute of Mental Measurements. • Years covered: 1989–present. Earlier *Mental Measurements Yearbooks* are available in print, published irregularly since 1938. • Access by subscription.	*http://www.unl.edu/buros/*	Contains descriptive information and reviews of English-language standardized tests covering educational skills, personality, vocational aptitude, psychology, and related areas as included in the print version of *Mental Measurements Yearbooks.* Often referred to as "Buros," after its longtime editor the late Oscar Buros.
National Institute of Nursing Research • Free Web site.	*http://www.nih.gov/ninr/*	The institute has a mandate to support clinical and basic research "to establish a scientific basis for the care of individuals across the life span—from management of patients during illness and recovery to the reduction of risks for disease and disability, the promotion of healthy lifestyles, promoting quality of life in those with chronic illness, and care for individuals at the end of life." The site includes links to conferences and events, research training, funding and programs.
National Nursing Quality Indicators Database	*http://www.nursingworld.org/quality/costing.htm*	Sponsored by the American Nurses Association, NQI is creating a national database to model patient outcomes. The database will provide a statistical modeling of care indicators and patient adverse outcomes, including costs, charges, length of stay, and adverse outcomes.
Nursing Studies Index, prepared by Yale University School of Nursing Index Staff under the direction of Virginia Henderson, RN, MA. Philadelphia: Lippincott, 1963–1972.		Annotated index to reported studies, research methods, historical and biographical materials in periodicals, books, and pamphlets in English. In 4 volumes: v. 1. 1900–1929, v. 2. 1930–1949, v. 3. 1950–1956, v. 4. 1957–1959.

TABLE 3.1 *(continued)*

Resource/Publisher	URL	Description
PsycINFO® Washington, D.C.: American Psychological Association. • Updated: weekly. • Access by individual or institutional subscription. • Years covered: 1872–present.	*http://www.apa.org*	Bibliographic database contains citations and summaries of journal articles, book chapters, books, dissertations, and technical reports, all in the field of psychology and the psychological aspects of related disciplines. Journal coverage includes international material selected from more than 1,500 periodicals written in over 35 languages. Current chapter and book coverage includes worldwide English-language material published from 1987–present.
Science Citation Index Philadelphia, PA: Thomson ISI® (founded as the Institute for Scientific Information®). • Updated: weekly. • Years covered: 1945–present • Access by subscription.	*http://www.isinet.com/ isi/*	Access to current and retrospective bibliographic information, author abstracts, and cited references found in more than 5900 science and technical journals, covering more than 150 disciplines, including medicine and nursing, informatics, and bioethics. Cited reference searching allows the searcher to track articles forward to journals that have cited a book or another article.
Social Sciences Citation Index Philadelphia, PA: Thomson ISI® (founded as the Institute for Scientific Information®). • Updated: weekly. • Years covered: 1956–present. • Access by subscription.	*http://www.isinet.com/ isi/*	Bibliographic database for more than 1,725 journals across 50 social sciences disciplines, selected, relevant items from over 3,300 of the world's leading scientific and technical journals. Cited reference searching allows the searcher to track articles forward to journals that have cited a book or another article.
Sociological Abstracts San Diego, CA: Sociological Abstracts. • Updated: monthly. • Years covered: 1963–present. Print equivalent: *Sociological Abstract,* 1952–1963. • Access by subscription.	*http://mdl.csa.com/csa/ factsheets/socioabs. shtml*	Bibliographic database for the international literature in sociology and related disciplines in the social and behavioral sciences. Abstracts of journal articles and citations to book reviews drawn from over 1,700 serials publications, and abstracts of books, book chapters, dissertations, and conference papers. Of interest to nursing, subject areas include family and social welfare, health, medicine and law, social development, social psychology and group interaction, substance abuse and addiction, welfare services, and women's studies.

(continued)

TABLE 3.1 *(continued)*

Resource/Publisher	URL	Description
Sigma Theta Tau International, and Virginia Henderson Electronic Library Indianapolis, IN: Sigma Theta Tau International. • Access is complimentary on the web.	*http:// www.stti.iupui.edu/ VirginiaHendersonLibrary/*	Links to databases including the Registry of Nursing Research, Nursing Knowledge Indexes, and Research Data Sets, and the Online Journal of Knowledge Synthesis for Nursing, an evidence-based, peer reviewed source. The Literature Index covers the nursing journals in which 50% or more articles are research articles and dates back to 1996. The Registry of Nursing Research (RNR) contains information and abstracts from over 16,000 studies. Research findings are indexed by variables or phenomenon of study as well as by researcher, title of the study, or keywords provided by the researchers. Studies are not peer reviewed for quality. It is up to the individual registrant to provide enough information about his or her work to allow the users to make their determinations of relevance and quality.
Trip Database Plus • Search tool freely available on the internet, with links to free abstracts and selected full text.	*http:// www.tripdatabase.com/*	TRIP (Turning Research Into Practice) brings together evidence-based healthcare resources available on the Internet, including systematic reviews, clinical guidelines, peer-reviewed journals, and more. Includes a feature that allows saved searches and clinical area alerting by email.

As bibliographic indexes have migrated to web-based electronic format, strategies for filtering the vast body of literature have emerged with the advent of "evidence-based" practice, which uses methodology-based criteria to identify the best information.

A. Primary Source Databases

Databases use standard controlled vocabulary terms (e.g., "MESH" terms or "subject headings") that describe the literature by topic as well as by research design. Controlled vocabulary terms may differ among databases; searchers should consult print or online thesauri to determine correct indexing terms: for example, "Hispanics" in PsycINFO or "Hispanic Americans" in Medline. Article types such as "clinical trial" or "systematic review" enable the end user of electronic databases to construct a search strategy to filter these studies from the published literature, retrieving a higher level of evidence that may be suitable for clinical decision making. Although research evidence remains an important component of evidence-based practice, a model for evidence-based decision making in nursing considers clinical expertise, patient preferences, and qualitative information that may override a treatment decision (DiCenso, Cullum, & Ciliska, 1998). Nursing's focus on qualitative research challenges the searcher to use alternative approaches to capture the evidence in the literature that is not easily measured. Strategies for filtering the literature by criteria such as phenomenology, ethnographic research, "lived experience," and other research designs have been described (Edward G. Miner Library, University of Rochester Medical Center, 2003).

B.   Secondary Source Databases

In addition to the primary source material in an original journal article, secondary sources synthesize and critically appraise research in review articles, systematic reviews, meta-analyses, and abstract journals such as *Evidence Based Nursing* (BMJ Publishing Group Ltd.). The Cochrane Collaboration is described below as an example of an international effort to update systematic reviews of the health care literature and disseminate this information (Cochrane Collaboration, 2003). Clinical practice guidelines are another source of secondary, pre-evaluated information based on research. The National Guideline Clearinghouse (http://www.guideline.gov/), produced by the Agency for Healthcare Research and Quality (AHRQ), is a searchable database of clinical guideline resources that synthesize research for healthcare professionals.

C.   Fee-Based Databases

A search of the peer-reviewed scholarly literature of nursing is best begun searching databases that organize citations in a consistent way. Most of these databases are fee-based (accessible via individual or institutional license), not free on the Internet. Following up on the initial database search and accessing the full text of research studies will require access to the resources of an academic health sciences library. A small percentage of the scholarly literature may be accessed on the free web, but a comprehensive search cannot be undertaken using search engines that randomly collect information that is arranged in a nonstandard way.

Table 3.1 lists a selection of electronic and print indexes for researching the nursing and allied health journal literature, including secondary resources with pre-evaluated information. Most of the sources are listed as available via subscription. Consulting with library staff is recommended to find the best way to access resources licensed by institutions as well as to take advantage of training.

VI.   ALTERING SERVICES

Many database services and individual journal publishers offer "alerting" or current awareness services. Researchers may create a profile to set up a topic or table of contents alert when an article or journal is published. Profiles may be set up by author, topic, or keywords. Electronic alerts may be created (often free with registration) by journal packages such as that offered by Science Direct (http://www.sciencedirect. com/), abstract journals such as *Evidence Based Nursing* (http://ebn.bmjjournals.com/ cgi/alerts/etoc), or many other individual journal publishers. Electronic discussion groups for many nursing specialties are also available (HealthWeb, 2002).

VII. BIBLIOGRAPHIC MANAGEMENT TOOLS

Software programs, such as EndNote, Reference Manager, Procite (all from Thompson ISI ResearchSoft, Carlsbad, CA), or Refworks (Refworks, Encinitas, CA), are invaluable tools for building a personal database of references; organizing them by subject, author, or other criteria; and citing the literature in a standard style format. The results of searches from bibliographic databases, online catalogs, and the results of alerting services may be downloaded into a personal database, customized to the user. Descriptors may be added to records, along with reading notes and other relevant links; all data is then searchable. Bibliographic management software is used in conjunction with word-processing software to cite references in text, create footnotes and endnotes, and output reference lists in standard formats.

4

Theoretical and Conceptual Frameworks

The body of literature on nursing theories, conceptual models, and nurse theorists is abundant. Works by Peggy Chinn, Maeona Kramer, Julia George, Jaqueline Fawcett, Leslie Nicoll, Joyce Fitzpatrick, Ann Whall, Lorraine Walker and Kay Avant, and Afaf Meleis, to name but a few, describe not only the existing nursing theories but also the development, analysis, and evaluation of theories and conceptual models in nursing. Readers are encouraged to refer to these references for a more extensive treatment of these topics.

I.   In the process of identifying and defining the research question, the researcher uses the vast resources of the world of literature, as previously described. The process of review is determined to a great extent by the type of research, whether the method is qualitative or quantitative or a combination of the two.

II.   RESEARCH CONCEPTS (QUANTITATIVE)

In the preliminary stages of review, the researcher determines what is known about the concepts to be studied. This process includes an identification of the concepts or theory underlying the research area. The literature review can provide vast amounts of information that can prove daunting to a novice researcher, particularly given the voluminous amounts of electronic data available. Therefore careful scrutiny and skills in using the tools for searching electronic databases are essential. Very often the researcher will either perform a cursory review or too broad a search or else become immersed in an examination of the minutiae of some findings. Repetitive search efforts and the assistance of a knowledgeable health sciences librarian will help immeasurably. The availability and access to large electronic data sets, although vast, have improved the process and quality of the research process.

Once the concepts have been identified, the underlying theory or conceptual framework is defined. This "proof of concept" will form the basis for the research and provide direction for the methodology. In establishing a theoretical framework a series of propositions regarding the interrelationships among concepts are identified. The goal of quantitative research is to test a theory or support a conceptual framework. The literature review should focus on defining the concepts within the theoretical framework and supporting relationships among the concepts/constructs to generate research questions or hypotheses. The identified concepts support the phenomena under study. The interaction of phenomena, theory, and concepts is essential. A thorough review of the literature assists the researcher in abstracting the concepts or constructs to be studied; this process may require a number of iterations and reflections on the phenomena under study. By the process of deduction the researcher then formulates a set of propositions that becomes the foundation of the research and results in the development of the hypothesis or research question. Familiarity with the literature is essential to this process.

III. RESEARCH CONCEPTS (QUALITATIVE)

The qualitative researcher approaches the process of the literature review in a different manner than does the quantitative researcher. The researcher's familiarity with the literature is important, but the approach is more flexible than in quantitative research in that the researcher does not usually identify a theory in the beginning of the research process, but rather focuses on building theory or generating hypotheses as a product of the research; it is a more inductive approach. The electronic tools available to the qualitative researcher include case studies of clients and consumers in large databases, such as the Cochrane Collaboration. These datasets can enhance the researcher's observations and reflections on themes and phenomena. Additionally, the qualitative researcher now has access to qualitative tools and software for identifying themes and clustering narrative information during data analysis. Examples of this type of software are Nudist and HyperResearch. A thorough discussion of qualitative principles can be found in Chapter 5 on Research Designs.

IV. FRAMEWORKS (QUANTITATIVE)

A. Definition of a Framework

1. Conceptual underpinnings of a study.
2. Not every study is based on a theory or conceptual model, but every study has a framework.
3. "In a study based on a theory, the framework is referred to as the *theoretical framework*; in a study that has its roots in a specific conceptual model, the framework is often called the *conceptual framework*" (Polit & Hungler, 1999, p. 110).

B. Conceptual Framework

1. Provides different perspectives or frames of reference for the phenomena of interest.

2. Is more abstract than theories
3. Provides "focus which directs the questions one asks and the theories one proposes and subsequently tests. It provides a network within which questions, theories, and data fit together and make possible the identification of needed areas of theory development" (Margaret Newman, quoted in Fawcett, 1993, p. 20).

C. Theory/Theoretical Framework

1. Composed of concepts that are more concrete than those in a conceptual framework, although conceptual frameworks influence theory development.
2. Relationships between the concepts in a theoretical framework may be specific, which provides the theoretical framework for quantitative research.
3. Quantitative investigators can base research on a theory in several ways. The most common approach is to test hypotheses deduced from a previously proposed theory.

D. Overview of Theoretical Frameworks (Quantitative)

1. Theory

    a. A series of propositions regarding the interrelationships among variables from which a large number of empirical observations can be deduced
    b. A systematic explanation of some phenomenon, broader and more complex than a fact
    c. Identifies the variables needed to explain the phenomenon and suggests the nature of the relationships between the variables
    d. Often generates one or more hypotheses to be tested (by deductive logic)

2. Proposition

    a. A statement indicating a relationship
    b. A set of propositions must form a logically interrelated deductive system (e.g., the theory composed of propositions must provide a mechanism for logically arriving at new statements from the original propositions)

3. Axioms

    a. Causal assumptions having the property of a directional relationship: "Select as axioms those propositions that involve variables that are taken to be directly linked causally" (Blalock, 1969). Axioms should therefore be statements that imply direct causal links among variables" (Dubin, 1969.)

4. Variables (see pp. 5–6)
5. Concept

    a. A word that expresses an abstraction formed by generalization from particulars (inductive logic)

6. Construct

    a. A concept
    b. Consciously invented or adapted for a scientific purpose

E. Overview of Theoretical Frameworks (Qualitative)

1. Purpose

There are contrary views regarding the use of a theoretical framework prior to data collection. Using a primarily inductive process, qualitative approaches are used to generate hypotheses and theory rather than test theory. The theory should emerge from the investigation. The conceptualizations that are developed are grounded in the actual observations and narratives of the participants.

2. Examples of Appropriate Frameworks

If a theoretical perspective is used, it must conform to the philosophical orientations and underpinnings of qualitative research. Examples of appropriate frameworks are:

    a. Phenomenology
    b. Symbolic interaction
    c. Culture
    e. History
    f. Aesthetics
    g. Hermeneutics
    h. Chaos theory
    i. Ecological psychology
    j. Heuristics
    k. Ethics
    l. Constructivism
    m. Postmodernism
    n. Poststructuralism
    o. Relational/co-construction

V.   DEFINITIONS OF VARIABLES (QUANTITATIVE)

    A.   There can be no scientific research without observations, and observations are not possible without clear and specific instructions on what and how to observe.

        1.   Serve as bridges between the theory-hypothesis level and the level of observation
        2.   Enable the researcher to measure variables

    B.   Both conceptual and operational definitions are important

        1.   Conceptual definition

            a.   A definition that defines a construct with other constructs
            b.   A variable may be defined by using other words
            c.   A variable may be defined by specifying what actions or behaviors the variable expresses or implies

        2.   Operational definition

            a.   A definition that assigns meaning to a construct or a variable by specifying the activities or operations necessary to measure the construct or variable

VI.   DEFINITIONS (QUALITATIVE)

In qualitative research, there are no a priori definitions of the phenomenon under study. Definitions emerge from the inquiry as themes, descriptions of the phenomenon, depictions of meaning, and/or portrayals of experiences. In Grounded Theory, definitions of the theoretical concepts and their relationships are an outcome of the study.

5

Research Designs

The issue of which design is appropriate to answer a particular research question is relatively complex. Within the "rough" categories of "quantitative" and "qualitative" designs are many designs with specific characteristics. A basic understanding of these characteristics is important to selecting a design that (1) has the potential for answering the research question, (2) is relatively precise and efficient, and (3) will produce valid and reliable results.

Research designs vary with regard to how much structure the researcher imposes on the research situation. "In a typical quantitative study, the researcher specifies the nature of any intervention, the nature of the comparisons, the methods to be used to control extraneous variables, the timing of data collection, the study site and setting, and the information to be given to participants" (Polit & Hungler, 1999, p. 160). In a qualitative study, there is no attempt to control predetermined variables or conditions as the inquiry is open to what emerges naturally in real life situations. The design is flexible and emphasizes discovery.

The major characteristics of quantitative and qualitative designs are discussed in this chapter. Quantitative research designs often involve comparisons that may be classified as *within-subjects* or *between-subjects* comparisons. The comparison to be made is indicated in the hypothesis. The factor of time is important. *Cross-sectional* designs involve the collection of data at one point in time, whereas *longitudinal* designs are intended to collect data at more than one point in time. Another distinction, in terms of quantitative designs, is *prospective* versus *retrospective* designs. A nonexperimental prospective design begins with presumed causes linked longitudinally to the presumed effect.

Most research is expensive in terms of time, effort, and possibly funds. Thus it is essential that the design be selected and implemented with care. The standards for both quantitative and qualitative designs are rigorous. If these issues are not taken seriously, the investigator may (1) encounter costly problems in the study, (2) be unable to complete the research, or (3) not know how to report the findings.

I.   THE RESEARCH DESIGN

The research design provides a plan that governs the conduct of the research and is a function of the research question(s) to be answered. Research questions may generate from nursing practice, an existing theory, a theoretical framework developed from the scientific literature, conceptual models, the literature, or human and social issues.

A.   Types of research designs (quantitative)

    1.   Descriptive
    2.   Experimental
    3.   Quasi-experimental
    4.   Correlational

B.   Types of research designs (qualitative)

    1.   Phenomenology
    2.   Grounded theory
    3.   Ethnography
    4.   Case study
    5.   Historiography
    6.   Hermeneutics
    7.   Ethnomethodology
    8.   Critical/emancipatory research
    9.   Action research
    10.   Foundational inquiry/philosophical analysis
    11.   Reflexivity
    12.   Aesthetics
    13.   Biography/life history/oral history

II.   THE RESEARCH DESIGN (QUANTITATIVE)

A.   Characteristics/aims of the quantitative design

    1.   Descriptive

        a.   Obtain information on topics for which there is little previous investigation
        b.   Describe events as they exist naturally
        c.   No introduction of anything new
        d.   No modification or control of the situation being studied

    2.   Experimental

        a.   Determine whether or not a predicted result occurs when a specified action is taken
        b.   Conducted under a controlled situation

— some factors are held constant
— other factors are manipulated
— random sampling and assignment to groups
— the results in the manipulated situation are evaluated and compared with those observed in the controlled situation

3. Quasi-experimental

a. Attempt to approximate a true experimental design when certain essential characteristics of a true experimental design cannot be attained; for example, the researcher is not able to:

— randomly sample
— manipulate factors
— control when or to whom the experimental treatment will be introduced

4. Correlational

a. Exploration of relationships among variables
b. Regression studies are a special case of correlational designs

— the researcher attempts to explain or predict changes in one variable (criterion) on the basis of changes in the other factors (predictors)

B. Sampling in quantitative designs (see chapter 6)
C. Measurement in quantitative designs (see chapters 7 and 8)
D. Protection of human subjects

1. Discuss the nature of participation in the study, and reinforce by a written description
2. Assure that consent or refusal will not affect health care (if appropriate)
3. Explain procedures for assurance of confidentiality or anonymity
4. State that withdrawal from the study at any time is permitted without repercussions
5. Develop a mechanism by which results of the study will be provided

III. THE RESEARCH DESIGN (QUALITATIVE)

A. Characteristics of qualitative research designs/approaches: There are a variety of designs/approaches in qualitative research. Following are descriptions of some of the more common ones and "central questions" (Patton, 1990, p. 88) that the approach raises.

1. Phenomenology

    a. Involves understanding the essence of a phenomenon
    b. Describes the "lived experience" from the perception of those experiencing it
    c. Asks "What is the structure and essence of experience of this phenomenon for these people?"
    d. Emanates from phenomenological philosophy
    e. For example: *The experience of alienation in nursing home residents: A phenomenological inquiry*

2. Grounded Theory

    a. Develop or generate a theory grounded in/derived from empirical data to explain a phenomenon or social/psychological process
    b. Emanates from sociology/symbolic interactionism
    c. For example: *Negotiating in interdisciplinary teams: A grounded theory*

3. Ethnography

    a. Study of cultures and "life ways" of people
    b. Asks "What is the culture of this group of people?"
    c. Emanates from social and behavioral sciences
    d. For example: *Bodymindspirit: Understanding the culture of holistic practitioners*

4. Case Study

    a. A holistic, detailed, and in-depth exploration of an individual, group as an entity, an organization, or an event in context, conducted in natural, real-life situations. Emanates from social and behavioral sciences
    b. For example: *The family experience with multiple births: A case study*

5. Historiography

    a. Investigates, analyzes, interprets, and narrates past events through a critical examination and synthesis of historical evidence such as documents, artifacts, personal accounts
    b. Emanates from history
    c. For example: *A history of the NYU Division of Nursing from 1960–1975*

6. Hermeneutics

    a. The art of interpretation in context so that text, human acts, or outcomes can be understood

b. Asks "What are the conditions under which a human act took place or a product was produced that make it possible to interpret its meaning?"
c. Emanates from philosophy, theology, and literary criticism
d. For example: *The language of caring in the nursing literature: A hermeneutical analysis*

7. Ethnomethodology

   a. Focus on people's understandings, the routine of the common social world
   b. Asks "How do people make sense of their everyday activities so as to behave in socially acceptable ways?"
   c. For example: *A study of the meaning of life in a wheelchair*

8. Critical or emancipatory research

   a. Attempts to surface and expose injustice and oppression within the context of the empowerment and emancipation of people
   b. Emanates from critical theory and postmodern social theory
   c. For example: *Hidden lives: Giving voice to sexually abused adolescents*

9. Action Research

   a. Practice oriented research that is conducted in collaboration with participants in a program, organization, or community
   b. Incorporates data collection and problem identification, planning, implementing and evaluating changes to solve problems and improve a specific system
   c. Emanates from social and action theory
   d. For example: *Funded research on women's health problems: Inquiry for change*

10. Foundational inquiry or philosophical analysis

    a. "Used to articulate, clarify, and refine basic conceptualizations" (Edgerton, 1988, p. 176)

       — done through philosophical analysis, a method of reflection and argumentation, leading to the "clarification of the language of a science" demonstrating the "possible reconciliation of apparently different concepts" (Manchester, 1986, p. 241), and reconceptualizations to increase the consistency between conceptual foundations or assumptions and particular scientific frameworks.

    b. For example: *A philosophical analysis of suffering*

11. Reflexivity

    a.   Critical reflection and awareness where the focus is on researchers' historical and geographic situation; their personal investment in the research; the perceptual, cognitive, theoretical, linguistic, political, and cultural biases they bring to the work; their "highs" and "lows" in the research endeavor (Gergen & Gergen, 2000; Alvesson & Kajskoldberg, 2000).

    b.   Being both researcher and participant: "The juxtaposition of self and subject matter is used to enrich the report . . . personal investments in the [research] act are not only recognized but become a subject of the research" (Gergen & Gergen, 2000, p. 1027).

    c.   "The interpretation of an interpretation and the launching of critical self-exploration of one's own interpretation of empirical material (including its construction)" (Alvesson & Kajskoldberg, 2000, p. 6)

    d.   Asks, "How has the researcher's subjectivity been both a producer and a product of this study?"

    e.   For example: *From interview to narrative; Living with cancer*

12. Aesthetics

    a.   Modes of research/representation using appreciation, and creative and artistic expression in understanding and representing meaning

    b.   Includes forms such as drama, performance, dance, music, film, paintings, photography, poetry, fiction, graphic art, video, multimedia

    c.   For example: *Surviving 9/11: Portrayals of firefighters through art*

13. Biography/life history/oral history (Cresswell, 1998)

    a.   Biography: Study of an individual and those experiences as told to the researcher or found in life documents and archival materials that describe important moments in an individual's life

    b.   Life history: Report on an individual's life and how it reflects cultural and societal themes, institutional themes, and social histories; a person's, group's, or organization's view of their lives in their own terms

    c.   Oral history: A person's recollections of events, their causes, and their effects, from the person or several other individuals either verbally, through tape recordings, or through writings.

    d.   These histories may be of individuals who have died or who are still living

    e.   For example: *The lady with the torch: Florence Nightingale—A Biography*

B.   Characteristics of the qualitative design

    1.   The design is flexible. It emerges as understanding increases; the specifics of the approach evolve as the inquiry proceeds.

2. The research process proceeds in a spiral, looping, cyclic fashion. Data collection and data analysis are blended, occur simultaneously, and inform one another.

3. The sample is usually small and emphasizes depth versus breadth.

4. The sample is chosen purposively or theoretically versus randomly or by convenience, and is selected serially (e.g., who and what comes subsequently depends on who and what came before).

5. There is a partner relationship between the researcher and the participant or "knower" of the phenomenon.

6. Two primary techniques are used in gathering data: participant observation and in-depth, unstructured interviewing. Other techniques include videotapes, photographs, projective techniques, life history, kinesics, and analysis of various documents.

7. Data are gathered over time. There is prolonged engagement in the field.

8. Data analysis focuses on discovery of patterns, description, and interpretation of the data to "make meaning."

9. Analysis and conclusions are directly supported by (grounded in) the actual data.

10. Qualitative analysis is usually presented in narrative rather than numerical form.

11. Qualitative inquiry necessitates a continuous and honest exploration of the researcher's own values and ethical orientations. During data collection, the researcher brackets preconceived notions, beliefs, attitudes, values, and knowledge about the phenomenon to "see" and "hear" the experience of the other.

C. Qualitative design or approach—general

1. Used to orient the reader, includes:

   a. Purpose of the approach
   b. Philosophical assumptions of the approach
   c. Background/foundation of the approach
   d. Definitions of the terms of the approach
   e. Process and procedures of the approach
   f. Result of the approach—what will it produce and why is this important in this study?

D. Qualitative design/approach—specific

1. This is the application of the specific design/approach as implemented in this study. It is a thorough explication of the details of this study.

   a. Repeat the purpose of the study and the research question

b.   Describe how each process will be carried out in this study (with the understanding that the design is flexible and may change as the inquiry progresses)

c.   Include a time line

E.   Sample—participants

1.   This is a description of the sample or unit of analysis (individual, group, culture, event or process).

a.   Describe the setting; give rationale for the setting

b.   Identify the sampling method (purposive/selective or theoretical) and describe sampling procedure

c.   Describe how entree to the setting, both official and informal, will be gained

d.   Describe how saturation will be achieved (continuation of sampling to the point of redundancy until no new or disconfirming information or evidence is found)

F.   Data Collection

In qualitative research the investigator is the research instrument, and as the primary data-gathering instrument can adjust and include the multitude and complexity of realities that s/he will encounter as a human being. The researcher can appreciate, understand and evaluate meanings that participants give to their experiences. Data for qualitative inquiries come from various sources: observations, interviews, verbal reports, documents, pictures, diaries, artifacts, and so on.

1.   Participant observation

a.   A period of intense interaction between the researcher and participants in the participants' setting. During this period, data are unobtrusively and systematically collected. The researcher is an involved observer, taking part in some activities while carefully observing the situation in order to record and analyze what is occurring.

b.   The researcher observes people, setting, atmosphere, activities, interactions/dialogue, events, context, and responses to the researcher.

c.   The researcher must consider the role of the observer, characterization of the researcher's role to others, depiction of the research purpose to others, duration of the observations, and focus of the observation (Patton, 1990).

d.   The researcher looks for who is present, what is happening, when activities occur, where they occur, why things happen, and how things happen.

e. Informal interviewing often is used for participant clarification, explanation, or expansion.

2. In-depth or unstructured interviewing

a. "A conversation with a purpose," which should produce interesting and prolific stories, data that are abundant in detail and examples, and narratives that reveal people's complex feelings, perceptions, and viewpoints.
b. The researcher should have an interview guide of 5 to 6 questions with which to begin the interview.
c. Questions may change as data are analyzed and other areas take on importance
d. Probe follow-up questions are used to increase more detailed inquiry
e. Use of a tape recorder to tape interviews

3. Prior to data collection identify and bracket or suspend one's assumptions, preconceptions, beliefs, attitudes, values, perspectives, and knowledge about the phenomenon under study in order to see, know, and understand the phenomenon or experience of the participants. This process of bracketing is also known as epoche.

4. Discuss the details and procedures of data gathering techniques (e.g., how conducted, when, where, with whom, approximate time per data collection sessions, use of tape recorder, transcriber, etc.)

5. Describe the data records to be used for the study

a. Field notes—detailed recordings of a variety of information (setting, dialogue, activities, events, feeling tone, etc.) collected in the field. These can be both descriptive and reflective.
b. Interview transcripts
c. Personal/methodological journal—the personal/methodological notes taken during the inquiry, including the researcher's ideas about the project, uniqueness of the method, methodological issues and how they were handled, and the researcher's feelings about the study, participants, assumptions, reactions, and the researcher's frame of mind at the time
d. Analytic log—the researcher's theoretical notes, analytic memos, and conceptualizations over the course of the inquiry, including interpretations, conjectures, inferences, and speculations about what is being learned and the emerging patterns, themes, and concepts

6. Discuss how and where the data will be stored
7. Discuss anticipated problems in data collection and the potential researcher's effect on the design

G. Protection of human subjects

    1. Discuss informed consent and how confidentiality of the participants is to be ensured. Anonymity cannot usually be assured in qualitative research due to the nature of the process.
    2. Address human subjects' review both at the university and, if indicated, at the settings in which the study will take place
    3. Consider potential ethical dilemmas when observing or interviewing about sensitive topics
    4. Identify referral sources if the nature of the inquiry may be potentially upsetting to the participant
    5. Consider how negotiations will be handled

III. TRIANGULATED DESIGNS

A. The use of multiple methods when studying the same phenomenon to potentially increase the reliability, validity, or comprehensiveness of a research study. A means of checking the inferences, assertions, hypotheses, or theory one draws by examining a single phenomenon from more than one vantage point or perspective.

B. Data triangulation

    1. The use of more than one data source or sampling strategy in a study (e.g., interviewing/observing a number of participants/settings about the same phenomenon, or "sampling" the same participant repeatedly over time)

C. Investigator triangulation

    1. Use of multiple researchers (interviewers, observers, coders, analysts) in the same study (e.g., team research)

D. Theoretical triangulation

    1. The use of several different theoretical perspectives or frames of reference in the analysis of the same set of data collected in the study

E. Methodological triangulated designs (mixed/multimethod/blended)

    1. Within method: Use of two or more data collection techniques within the same methodological approach/tradition (e.g., interviewing and participant observation and participant journaling in a grounded theory study)
    2. Between or across method: use of two or more different or dissimilar methodological approaches/traditions (e.g., quantitative and qualitative designs in the same research study)

IV. FACTORS AFFECTING THE SELECTION OF A RESEARCH DESIGN

    A.   The research question(s)

        1.   Generally, there are several designs that can be employed in studying a given broad research problem.
        2.   Alternative designs that are equally valid for investigating a problem are rarely equally efficient.

    B.   Knowledge of the research topic
    C.   Knowledge of different kinds of designs
    D.   Application of criteria for selecting a design

        1.   Has the potential for answering the research question (and testing the hypotheses in the case of a quantitative design)
        2.   Relatively precise and efficient
        3.   Affords utilization of powerful statistical procedures if the design is *quantitative*
        4.   Economical for both the researcher and subjects/participants
        5.   Produces valid and reliable results
        6.   Allows an opportunity for comparison of study findings with the results of other investigations
        7.   Conforms to accepted procedures used in research on the designated topic

V.   QUANTITATIVE DESIGNS—INTERNAL AND EXTERNAL VALIDITY

In research, the researcher attempts to determine if the variable studied is actually the "causal" factor or if there are extraneous or intervening variables unaccounted for in the study setting. In other words, in studying the relationship between an independent and a dependent variable, one is hypothesizing that the independent variable is related to the occurrence of the dependent variable. But is "X" always the factor that operates in the occurrence of "Y" or is there an extraneous, or intervening, variable confounding the situation?

Internal validity addresses the question of whether the researcher is measuring what s/he thinks s/he is. External validity is the extent to which the researcher can then make a generalization about the relationships identified in the experimental setting. Internal validity is achieved primarily by means of a good research design with maximum controls. External validity is more difficult to achieve than internal validity because subjects usually cannot be selected at random from a defined population.

For example: Is pre-operative structured teaching truly related to postoperative recovery or are there factors other than teaching playing a role in the results?

Note: A discussion of the design and methods for control of extraneous variables for this study may be found in Appendix D (pp. 176–182).

A.   Threats to validity

Source	Definition
History	—the effect of events that occur simultaneously with the investigation
Maturation	—changes in the subject as the result of conditions, such as fatigue
Regression toward the mean	—a group chosen because of its extreme position on a continuum will tend to exhibit movement toward the mean on retest
Testing	—the effect of one test on a subsequent test as the result of practice, memory, or training
Instrumentation	—the effect of variations in accuracy or efficiency of an instrument from time to time or from one condition to another
Differential selection of subjects	—selection of two or more groups that are not comparable on some crucial variable that may bias the outcome
Subject mortality	—the effect of differential losses from groups so that the final result is to render them not comparable

B.   Strategies for control

1.   In developing the theoretical rationale, consider the dependent variable and try to identify other variables that are related to it.
2.   Control the variables that are not under study but that may contribute substantially to the variance in the dependent variable(s).
3.   Maximize the experimental variable (e.g., make sure it will operate).
4.   Consider selecting a sample that controls for the extraneous variables (e.g., a sample that is homogeneous for those variables).
5.   Use random selection and/or random assignment for experimental and quasi-experimental designs whenever possible.

   a.   True randomization permits one to say that experimental groups are equal at the outset (e.g., it theoretically controls for extraneous variables)
   b.   Although randomization cannot always be achieved, care needs to be taken in assessing the similarity of groups

6.   An extraneous variable may be built into the design (e.g., measured, permitting the calculation of variance in the dependent variable that may be attributed to the variable).
7.   Subjects in the control and experimental groups may be matched for specific variables.
8.   Control the testing situation
9.   Minimize errors of testing.

6

Sampling Methods:
Basic Issues and Concepts

I. INTERNAL AND EXTERNAL VALIDITY OF QUANTITATIVE STUDIES

As noted, internal validity is whether or not the results of a specific quantitative study are accurate for the sample used in the investigation. External validity is whether or not valid sample results can be generalized to the larger population from which the sample was taken. They depend on the problem formation, measurement, statistical analysis, and sampling design.

A. Sampling principles and concepts

   1. Developed most fully within the tradition of survey research
   2. Experimental designs depend more on relatively small, convenience, or sometimes purposive samples due to

      a. Unavailability of large numbers of representative, willing subjects
      b. Practicality of administering treatments to large numbers of subjects
      c. Need for random assignment of subjects from the available sample pool to either an experimental or control group, thereby equating the two groups

   3. Quasi-experimental designs pose even greater strains on the principles of proper sampling

      a. Internal and external validity are more difficult to assess
      b. Experimenter frequently has no control over

         — the source of subjects
         — the size of the sample

— whether the subjects are in the experimental or control group
— the nature and administration of the treatment

For further study of the basic topics presented in this chapter as well as other advanced aspects of sampling, see Dillman (1999), Groves et al. (2001), Lohr (1999), and Scheaffer (1996).

II. SAMPLING ERROR AND SAMPLING BIAS

   A. Sampling error

      1. Deviations from true population parameters (e.g., population means, standard deviations, percentages, correlations, that result from the study of just one sample taken from that population)
      2. Probable error despite the fact that the sample was scientifically drawn
      3. Can be estimated
      4. A direct function of the size of a *properly* drawn sample
      5. Within limits, the larger the sample drawn, the smaller the probable error

   B. Sample bias

      1. Difficult to estimate in advance largely due to

         a. The way in which a sample is selected
         b. Whether the subjects fully cooperate

      2. Methods for avoidance

         a. Draw a *representative* sample
         b. Strive for as much cooperation as possible

            Ex. Low sample returns (if a mail questionnaire is used) or low sample cooperation (if phone or in-person interviews are conducted) signal that the sample statistics deviate in critical ways from the true population values.

III. FIVE LEVELS OF SAMPLING REALITY AND THEIR POTENTIAL IMPACT ON INTERNAL AND EXTERNAL VALIDITY

   A. Identifying the ideal population of interest

      1. Directly connected to a research problem (e.g., practicing nurses or hospital patients)

   B. Delimiting a subpopulation

1. The sample seldom remains at a general level (e.g., delimitations are either consciously stated or implicit)

   Ex. Patients who are males suffering from cancer and are in a hospice care setting

2. Insufficient delimitation leads to both unacceptable sampling error and bias

C. Locating a sampling frame

   1. Should be a fair reflection of the delimited population
   2. Sample from that frame by using some proper procedure such as simple random sampling or systematic sampling
   3. Available sampling frame may not reflect the desired population as delimited, leading to sample bias

D. Drawing the sample

   1. Some, if not many, of the subjects in the selected sample may fail to cooperate
   2. Sample size may be inadequate, leading to

      a. Larger than acceptable sampling error

E. Studying the sample

   1. Sample size may be less representative than the one originally drawn, leading to

      a. Potential sample bias

   2. Sample returned may be too small a proportion of that drawn and contacted, leading to

      a. Unacceptable sampling error
      b. Sample bias

IV. SAMPLING SOURCES OF FRAMES, STYLES OF SAMPLING, AND SAMPLE SIZE

A. Sources and availability of sampling frames

   1. Depends on the delimited population as specified by the research design

      Exs. — membership lists of social groupings
      — work rosters of organizations that contain the names of persons who fit the delimited population

2. Information about the sampling units are preferable to those that contain simply names and addresses

    a. Permits comparison of subjects who cooperated with those who chose not to cooperate

    b. Sheds light on the possibility of sampling bias introduced by noncooperation and the extent to which the sample drawn is representative of the larger frame

B. Styles of sampling

  1. Simple random sampling

    a. Basic approach upon which statistical significance testing and the assessment of confidence intervals are based

    b. Tests of statistical significance (e.g., the *t*-test, the *F*-test or chi square) indicate how frequently the results obtained from a study occur by chance

    c. Based on sample statistics, a confidence interval indicates the range of scores within which the true population value most probably falls

    d. Proper technique assures that all subjects in a sampling frame have an equal chance of being selected

    e. Every unit is assigned a number

    f. From a table of random numbers, subject IDs are selected until the desired number of units is reached

  2. Systematic sampling

    a. Every nth subject is taken from an unnumbered sampling frame until the desired quantity of subjects is selected

    b. Unacceptable if there are repeated patterns in the listing (e.g., names listed on each page are rank ordered in some way)

    c. Economical in terms of time

  3. Stratified sampling

    a. Assures *inclusion* of certain characteristics of a sample and/or *exclusion* of others

    b. Useful when the researcher wants to include certain characteristics in the sample in proportion to their presence in the larger population or disproportionately so

      Ex. If only males are to be studied, a sampling frame also containing females would have to be stratified according to gender and then limited to the selection of males only. If the males and females were to be compared, even though the researcher is sampling from a frame of elderly bedridden patients (usually composed of more females than males), then a disproportionately larger number of males and disproportionately smaller number of females would have to be selected in order to have an equal number of both sexes. If one were interested in certain matters related to the overall population of elderly, bedridden patients, then after stratifying according to gender, males and females would have to be selected in numbers proportionate to their presence in the larger elderly population. The selection within each stratum could be accomplished either by simple random sampling or systematically if the available list were in an unbiased form (e.g., alphabetical).

4.   Cluster sampling

a.   Used when there is an absence of an adequate frame for subjects

Ex.   In studying hospital nurses, one might have a list of hospitals in a certain area, but not the nurses within them. One way, therefore, to select nurses would be to select a few hospitals and then study all the nurses within them. Another would be to select hospitals, then floors within them, then study all the nurses on the selected floors.

5.   Quota sampling

a.   Useful when the research involves face-to-face interviews requiring the specification of a number of persons possessing particular characteristics (e.g., 20 females under 30 years of age who jog, 10 males over 40 who smoke, and

b.   When there is no clear sampling frame but a physical place where subjects can be located

Ex.   Interview of patients attending a particular clinic

6.   Snowball sampling

a.   Useful in situations where no actual sampling frame exists, and
b.   When few desired subjects are known
c.   The investigator starts with the few known subjects and from them attempts to connect with still others of the same kind until the desired sample size is reached

7.   Convenience sampling

    a.   Uses whatever cooperative subjects are easily at hand
    b.   Because of the way the subjects were selected, their representativeness is in question

C.   Sample size and methods to determine the minimum needed

    1.   General rules

        a.   For survey and correlational research, draw as large a sample as is financially possible, within certain limits
        b.   Generally, sample sizes larger than 1,000 to 1,200 subjects from populations of over 100,000 are unnecessary, as the increased accuracy of the statistics gained from larger samples does not justify the larger numbers and costs
        c.   Samples smaller than 200 or 300 subjects usually lead to confidence intervals that are too wide to be satisfying and also limit the kinds of subsample analyses that may be necessary

    2.   Methods to determine sample size

        a.   Power analysis if

           — the effect size can be specified
           — some judgment about sample variances can be made

        b.   Standard error formulas if

           — the researcher wants to be 95% sure that the true percentage or correlation falls within a limited range of plus or minus a few percentage points or correlational points

        c.   Rules of thumb

           — informal standards that over time have come to be accepted by professionals in various fields but typically are not easily traced back to their original sources

               Exs: — 20 to 30 subjects for each independent variable if the fundamental statistical analysis is to be multiple regression
                       — a minimum of 5 subjects for each item if factor analyses are to be done

      d.   Other factors

          — the greater the homogeneity of the population, the smaller the size of the sample needed

          — if the study is theory building, a smaller sample is required than if the purpose is theory testing or descriptive of a large population

          — the more variables and delimitations, the greater the need for larger numbers as comparisons of subgroups and combinations of variables necessitate larger numbers

          — if a sampling frame contains a large number of subjects who are no longer available, then a much larger number will be needed in order to reach the minimal size originally calculated

V. GENERAL SAMPLING SUGGESTIONS (QUANTITATIVE)

A.   Know as much as possible about the population and sampling frame.

B.   Find and use a sampling frame that is representative or clearly heuristic, given the research interest, that has more than names and addresses associated with it.

C.   Use sound sampling procedures (e.g., stratified random sampling).

D.   Within limits, draw as large a sample as is technically and financially feasible.

E.   Use follow-up procedures to achieve as high a return rate of questionnaires as possible or to gain the cooperation of phone or in-person interviewees.

VI. SAMPLING (QUALITATIVE DESIGNS)

A.   Qualitative research approaches often utilize small samples and emphasize depth versus breadth. The researcher is attempting to obtain understanding through an in-depth, information-rich, and detailed exploration of the phenomenon, group, or person.

B.   The sample is chosen purposively versus randomly or by convenience.

C.   The sample refers to the unit(s) of analysis to be explored such as an individual, a group, a culture, an organization or agency, an event or occurrence, a process, or a particular phenomenon that people experience.

D.   The sampling process necessitates an emphasis both on what to sample and how to sample.

E.   "The 'what' to sample may include events, places, persons, artifacts, activity, and time" (Kuzel, 1992, p. 34).

F.   The "how" to sample includes determining which of the various purposive sampling strategies to use.

      1.   Extreme or deviant case—highly unusual case

      2.   Intensity sampling—manifest phenomenon intensely (e.g., above/below average)

      3.   Maximum variation sampling—purposefully choosing a wide range of variation on dimensions of interest

4. Homogeneous sampling—focused, reduced variation
5. Typical case—highlights normal, average
6. Stratified purposeful sampling—particular subgroup of the population
7. Critical case—if true of this case, likely to be true of all other cases
8. Snowball or chain sampling—identify cases from people who know people etc.
9. Criterion sampling—cases that meet some criterion
10. Theory-based sampling—manifestation of a theoretical concept
11. Confirming and disconfirming cases—seeking exceptions, testing variations
12. Opportunistic sampling—following new or unexpected leads
13. Random purposeful sampling (still small sample size)—random within a purposeful category
14. Combination or mixed purposeful sampling—based on triangulation, multiple needs
   (Patton, 1990, pp. 182–183)

G. Theoretical sampling is used to generate grounded theory where the researcher decides on theoretical/analytic grounds what data to collect next and where to find them. What groups or subgroups of populations, events, activities (to find varying dimensions, strategies, etc.) does one turn to next in data collection? And for what theoretical purpose? The process of data collection is controlled by the emerging theory (Strauss and Corbin, 1998)

H. The researcher continues to sample individuals, events, situations, and/or settings to the point of redundancy or saturation where no new or disconfirming information or evidence is found.

7

Principles of Measurement

Measurement is an issue in any quantitative research. The spectrum of measurement extends from the directed interview to the highly structured, self-administered Likert scales that are scored. A full description of the many kinds of measurements, or observations, is beyond the scope of this book. Thus an outline of the principles of quantitative measurement is provided and the various kinds of measurement tools are described. These include the commonly used interviews and questionnaires, scales and other psychological measures, observational methods, and vignettes. Suggestions are provided for locating an appropriate measure for a study and assessing its validity and reliability. For a more comprehensive discussion of measurement issues, the reader is referred to the many texts on psychometric theory and measurement.

I. METHODS OF MEASUREMENT

    A.   Measurement consists of objective methods of observation

            1.   Those in which anyone following prescribed rules will assign the same ratings, or "scores," to what is observed
            2.   Agreement among observers is at a maximum
            3.   All methods of observation are inferential (e.g., inferences about attitudes or behaviors of individuals are made on the basis of the ratings assigned to items on specific forms of measurement instruments)

                    a.   Interviews and questionnaires
                    b.   Scales, tests, and other psychological measures
                    c.   Observational methods
                    d.   Vignettes

B.   Interviews and questionnaires

    1.   The interview

        a.   A direct method of obtaining information
        b.   May be used to study relationships and to test hypotheses
        c.   When used in research to test hypotheses

            — the questions, their sequence, and wording are fixed
            — the interview must be carefully constructed and pretested
            — the interview schedule must be subjected to the same criteria of reliability, validity, and objectivity as any other measuring instrument

    2.   The questionnaire

        a.   Differs from interviews in that they are self-administered and highly structured

C.   Scales and other psychological measures

    1.   The test

        a.   A systematic procedure in which the subject is presented with a set of items to which he or she responds
        b.   The examiner assigns a rating, or score, to each response
        c.   Inferences are made about the subject's possession of whatever the test is designed to measure
        d.   A trait, attitude, or emotion can be measured and quantified in this manner

    2.   The scale

        a.   A set of response symbols for each item that permits the assignment of a rating according to rules

            Ex.   Strongly agree   5
                     Agree   4
                     Undecided   3
                     Disagree   2
                     Strongly disagree

b. Assignment and totaling of the values or ratings indicates the degree to which the subject possesses the characteristic that the scale measures

c. Takes advantage of any intensity structure that may exist among the individual items

Ex. A measure of attitude toward research

Research is essential to the generation of new knowledge.

    SA   A   U   D   SD

Nursing research is a key factor in developing and evaluating practice.

    SA   A   U   D   D

Participation in conducting research is a responsibility of all members of the profession.

    SA   A   U   D   SD

Professional nurses should allocate time to research activities even if it requires use of free time.

    SA   A   U   D   SD

Presumably, if respondents agree with the content in one item, they are in agreement with all items preceding it in the list (e.g., those with lesser intensities).

D. Observational methods

1. A direct observation of behavior

   a. The investigator assigns values to behavioral acts, or sequences of acts, according to rules in order to obtain reliable and objective observations from which inferences may be drawn
   b. Requires an operational definition of what one is observing
   c. Behaviors must be assigned to categories that are mutually exclusive
   d. Units of behavior must be determined (molar versus molecular)
   e. Sampling, or when and how the observations will be made, must be decided (event sampling, time sampling)
   f. The nature of the relationship between the observer and subjects needs to be defined. Concealment refers to the degree to which subjects are aware that they are being observed; intervention means the degree to which the investigator structures the observational setting.

Ex. A study of exploratory behavior among children in relation to empathic behavior in parents. The investigator observes mothers and children interacting. A sequence of behaviors may be observed (e.g., the approach of child to mother, response of the mother, and reaction of the child).

II. GUIDES FOR LOCATING MEASUREMENT INSTRUMENTS

A. Know the nature of the variable to be studied
B. Consult good references on tests and measures
C. Search the periodical literature
D. Consult compiled reviews of measures
E. If no satisfactory measure is located, consider revision of an existing tool or construction of a new instrument

An excellent database of health and psychosocial instruments (HaPI) is published by the Behavioral Measurement Database Services (Perloff, 1996). The HaPI-CD permits access to 36,000 records of information on measurement instruments relevant to the health and psychosocial sciences. Available in Windows, the HaPI CD-ROM can be installed on any IBM-compatible PC with a CD-Rom drive, 640K RAM memory, and 500K free hard disk space.

III. ASSESSMENT OF VALIDITY AND RELIABILITY OF A MEASURE

A. Validity

1. Refers to whether an instrument or test actually measures what it is supposed to measure
2. Determined by

   a. Submitting the instrument to a group of judges or experts who estimate whether the *content* is representative of the universe of content of the characteristic being measured
   b. Checking to see if subjects are actually presently engaged in the activity or are able to exhibit the quality measured by the instrument (known as *concurrent* validity, similar to *predictive* validity)

      — often presented in the form of correlational data between the measurement and the outcome or between two measures that are purported to measure the same thing

    c.   Studying the relationship between the theory and the measurement of the constructs, or concepts, which make up the theory (known as *construct* validity)

    d.   Considering the construct definition for the measure and evaluating whether the items reflect that definition (known as *face* or *content* validity)

    e.   Comparing the responses to those of a group already known to have a particular characteristic or behavior

B.   Reliability

    1.   Refers to the proportion of accuracy to inaccuracy in measurement
    2.   Addresses the issue of stability (e.g., if a variable is measured repeatedly with the same or a comparable instrument will the same, or a similar, results be obtained?)
    3.   Determined by

    a.   *Test–retest*—a test is administered twice to the same subjects; if the test is reliable and the characteristic is stable, the results will be consistent

    b.   *Equivalent*—equivalent tests contain the same types of items based on the same material but the particular references and wording of items are different

    —   alternate forms of a test reveal a high correlation if tests are reliable

    c.   *Split-half*—compares the results of one-half of the items (odd numbered) to the other half (even numbered) on a measure—appropriate only if all the items are designed to measure the same construct

    —   a high correlation indicates reliability

    d.   *Statistical tests*—yield a reliability coefficient that is obtained by applying a statistical formula to the test scores

    Ex.   Kuder-Richardson
              Spearman Brown
              Cronbach's Alpha

e. *Item analysis*—a measure of internal consistency that examines the extent to which the whole test or scale is predictive of responses to individual items

— a high correlation between an item and the total score indicates the item is reliable

8

Development of Quantitative Measures

In recent years, there has been an enormous increase in the development of quantitative measures by nursing investigators. This trend has evolved in response to the interest in studying the human behaviors and responses that are of particular interest to nurses. Although this development is not surprising, as all research requires some form of observation or measurement, the sound psychometric principles developed in earlier years by other disciplines are applicable to the activities of nursing investigators. Thus the need for valid and reliable measures with a sound theoretical foundation led to the inclusion of this chapter.

The focus of this chapter is a relatively detailed description of the process used to develop a measure of need fulfillment in the partner relationship. Increasingly, nurses have become interested in the study of social support as a construct that plays a key role in the well-being of patients. The development of the Partner Relationship Inventory (PRI) occurred as a result of that interest. The continued development of the PRI has entailed the construction of alternate forms to measure change over time, both in patients and in families.

Nurses are in a prime position to interact with clients during the course of the different phases of an illness experience. Thus they frequently can evaluate needs as they vary over time and intervene in a timely and appropriate manner. The example of the development of the PRI is offered as an encouragement to those who may wish to join the challenge of developing measures that lend themselves to capturing change as it occurs in clients and families.

I. OBJECTIVES

   A. Create valid and reliable measures of behaviors and perceptions
   B. Different measures according to intended populations
   C. Test theory
   D. Construct alternate forms to capture change over time
   E. Develop culturally sensitive measures

II.   METHODOLOGICAL STEPS: CONSTRUCTION OF A MEASURE

    A.   Construct a theoretical framework, based on an exhaustive review of relevant literature

        Ex.   Hoskins, C. N. (1985). *The Partner Relationship Inventory*. Palo Alto, CA: Consulting Psychologists Press, Inc.

             The theoretical framework for the PRI was based on a review of literature from family theory, interpersonal conflict, and role theory. The framework is based on findings that indicate that interaction in family relationships is instrumental in fulfilling psychosocial needs of individual members. When the interaction is a true dialogue in which each participant first perceives, then complements the other's needs, the probability is greater that basic positive emotions will prevail and conflict will be minimal. Conversely, when the task of meeting specific psychosocial needs is not accomplished, conflict ensues.

    B.   Develop a construct definition

        Ex.   The construct definition for the PRI is: "the perceived degree of fulfillment of interaction and emotional needs." Studies of perceptual differences in partner relationships indicate that partners who perceive that they are not receiving responses from their mates in accordance with their expectations engage in provocative, domineering, and competitive behaviors that are conducive to conflict. Other investigations support the notion that perception is of crucial importance in the immediate outcome of the interaction, as well as in the fulfillment, or lack of fulfillment, of needs.

    C.   Construct the items

        Ex.   In early basic work (Mathews & Mihanovich, 1963), 400 items were constructed from an extensive review of the literature on conflict and classified into 50 problem areas distinguishing happy from unhappy relationships, 42% representing basic human needs and 36%, interactional needs. Permission was obtained to use the work in the development of the PRI.

        1.   The 50 items distinguishing happy and unhappy couples were placed in either the dimension of emotional or interactional need, depending on content.
        2.   The items were classified into eight categories reflecting a specific focus, five for the interactional need dimension and three for the emotional need dimension. (A fourth dimension was omitted because a varimax rotated factor analysis indicated it contributed to both dimensions.)
        3.   Each category was expanded to 10 items by formulating additional items with similar wording and essentially the same content.

4. Approximately half of the items were phrased in reverse form, facilitating the study of consistency in response and reduction in response set.

D. Arrange the total pool of items in a logical and smooth sequence, alternating the reverse-score items with positively phrased items.
E. Construct a response format, balancing positive and negative response options.
F. Submit the scale to selected experts for evaluation of items and response format using the following criteria:

1. Do the items represent the universe of content for the construct being measured, thus reflecting content validity?
2. Are the items appropriate for the designated population?
3. Are the items situation specific?
4. Do the items contain one idea rather than multiple ideas?
5. Are person and tense consistent?
6. Are there double negatives (e.g., are negative stems combined with negatively phrased options?)
7. What is the probability of response set? faking? social desirability?
8. Is the response format "balanced" (e.g., an equal number of positively and negatively phrased items?)
9. Are the instructions for respondents clear?
10. Do the instructions reflect whether the items are to be answered according to the moment (state) or in general (trait)?

G. Revise the scale, response format, and instructions according to the evaluations.
H. Select a valid and reliable measure for the study of construct validity of the newly constructed measure.

Ex. The Marital Adjustment Test (Locke & Wallace, 1959) was selected for construct validation of the PRI.

I. Submit the newly constructed measure, the selected measure for the study of construct validity, and a demographic form to a sample of appropriate size and characteristics.
J. Consider procedures to evaluate reliability (e.g., test-retest reliability requires respondents to complete the newly constructed measure at two designated times).

Ex. A sample of couples completed the PRI in both the morning and early evening.

K. Conduct preliminary preparation of the data.

1. Evaluate missing data
2. Reverse score items as indicated
3. Calculate subscale, or category, scores for all measures as indicated

L.   Estimate construct validity of the newly constructed measure.

    Ex.   Pearson product-moment correlation coefficients were calculated between the MAT total score and each PRI category score. The validity of the PRI was demonstrated to be moderate to high (range = .40–.75). Varimax rotated factor analyses provided a useful method for determining to what degree a category enhanced the measurement of fulfillment of needs in the interactional and emotional dimensions. The factor loadings for the categories on the appropriate dimension ranged from .63 to .91, thus verifying the theoretical structure of the scale.

M.   Estimate reliability

    Ex.   Pearson product-moment correlation coefficients between total scores for the categories and constituent items verified internal consistency. Pearson product-moment correlation coefficients between responses for the morning and evening for each category supported test-retest reliability (range = .84–.95).

N.   Temporal patterning

    1.   Nursing assessment and intervention necessitates multiple observations of behaviors over time. Qualitative and quantitative observations and measures facilitate

       a.   Definition of patterns in human behavior
       b.   Identification of change that occurs over time
       c.   Consideration of change in relation to other behaviors or constructs

          Ex.   Each of the morning and evening PRI category mean scores reflected an increase in negative feelings; however, the standard error of the difference between means for the morning and evening scores was significant for only two categories.

    2.   Construct alternate forms of a measure

       a.   A single observation of a defined behavior or interaction yields little information of value in terms of ongoing patterns within an individual or family system. Such study necessitates a sequence of observations of behaviors, perceptions, or feelings, either directly or by a measurement scale.

          Ex.   The method used to develop alternate forms of the PRI included the following steps:

1. For each category the means of the 10 items from the questionnaire completed early in the day were placed in rank order of magnitude.

Rank Ordering of Category 2 by Mean Values

Item	Mean
1	3.40
2	3.37
3	3.25
4	3.21
5	1.71
6	1.67
7	1.58
8	1.46
9	1.35
10	1.08

Items 1, 2, 3, and 4 are reverse-score items. The scores had not yet been reverse-scored, which is reflected in the magnitude of the mean values.

2. The 10 items were divided by the serpentine method into two groupings (e.g., the items were rank ordered according to mean values in serpentine pattern). The objectives were to

   a. Equalize groups in terms of expected degree of fulfillment as reflected in responses to items
   b. Achieve an approximately equal number of reverse-score items in each alternate form

Items in Category 2 Divided into Two Groups Using the Serpentine Method

	Group		
	A		B
Item	Mean	Item	Mean
1	3.40	2	3.37
4	3.21	3	3.25
5	1.71	6	1.67
8	1.46	7	1.58
9	1.35	10	1.08
Total	11.13		10.95

3. The means of Group A were added and compared to the total of the means of Group B

4. The means were approximately equal, indicating that the alternate forms would yield comparable scores

5. The procedure was repeated for each category and for both the inventory completed early in the day and the one completed late in the day

6. The four small groups within each category, consisting of a Group A and a Group B of both the early and late forms, were examined for level of reliability

7. The group means and standard deviations were calculated and the Pearson product-moment correlation coefficient was used to compute the group item, the interitem, and the intergroup correlation coefficients

8. The Spearman-Brown formula was used to determine the reliability levels of the groups by the split-half method

9. One alternate form of the scale was constructed by combining the five items from Group A of each of the categories into a 40-item scale. The second alternate form was constructed by combining the five items from Group B of each of the categories.

9

Data Analysis and Interpretation

The analyses and interpretation of data collected in quantitative and qualitative designs have significant differences. Both contribute a great deal to the knowledge base of nursing science, which has as a primary purpose excellence in patient care: Clearly, health care is increasingly influenced by the demand for universal access to care, cost containment, and public policy. As part of health care reform and managed care, outcomes of care that can be documented are receiving increased attention. Thus the findings and outcomes from nursing studies need to be evaluated for their potential to improve practice as well as for validity and credibility of their findings.

The purposes and processes of quantitative and qualitative data analyses are outlined in this chapter. Similar to the description of internal and external validity for quantitative designs in chapter 6, the criteria for quality, or rigor, in qualitative research are described. Whether the reader's purpose is to design a study or evaluate a study for application to practice, a basic knowledge of analyses and interpretation is essential for making such informed decisions.

I. DATA ANALYSIS AND INTERPRETATION (QUANTITATIVE DESIGNS)

   A. Statistical methods should be appropriate to the level of data collected. Interval and ordinal data are most often encountered in the behavioral sciences.
   B. Kinds of data

      1. Nominal

         a. Lowest level of measurement or means of classifying data
         b. Consists of classifying observations into categories

            — categories are mutually exclusive (e.g., each observation must be capable of classification into one and only one category)
            — any nominal variable may be dichotomized and then be treated as a binary variable, assigning a "1" to members of one group and a "0" to the other

2. Ordinal

    a. Distinguished from nominal data by the property of order among the categories

    b. Categories may be thought of as higher or lower than the adjacent category

    c. No specification of the magnitude of the interval between two categories

3. Interval

    a. Distinguished from ordinal data by having equal intervals between the units of measure (e.g., a score of 50 points is halfway between 40 and 60)

    b. A true quantitative score

    c. Lacks a true zero (e.g., one cannot interpret a score of 50 as indicating twice as much of a given trait or ability as 25)

4. Ratio

    a. Possesses all properties of interval scales

    b. Has a true zero

C. Nonparametric statistical procedures are indicated for nominal and ordinal data (e.g., chi square). Parametric statistics are intended for interval and ratio data (e.g., Pearson product–moment correlation coefficient).

D. Descriptive statistics (used to describe data). Descriptive statistics indicate the central tendency of scores (e.g., where the scores tend to group together) and the variability of scores (e.g., how far the scores spread from the center of the distribution of scores).

1. Measures of central tendency

    a. Mean

       — one of the most commonly used measures of central tendency

       — the arithmetic average of a set of data

$$\text{Mean} = \frac{\text{sum of } x}{n}$$

    b. Median

       — the midpoint in a set of highest to lowest ranked scores (e.g., the same number of scores are above the midpoint as below)

      —   if there is an even number of scores, the midpoint score is interpolated (e.g., a midpoint of 10 is interpolated for the set 5, 6, 7, 9, 11, 12, 12, 14 even though the score of 10 was not attained)

   c.   Mode

      —   consists of the most frequently occurring score in a distribution of scores
      —   usually located near the center of the distribution
      —   a less frequently used index of central tendency

2.   Guide to selection of measure of central tendency

   a.   Mean

      —   the only measure that uses all the data (e.g., all scores are used in computing the mean)
      —   provides the more sensitive index of central tendency
      —   more stable statistically
      —   when there are one or two extreme scores, however, the mean does not provide an accurate reflection of the average

   b.   Median

      —   not influenced by extreme scores
      —   a good index of central tendency when working with sets of data that depart from normal distributions (e.g., there is an extremely high proportion of superior scores and a low proportion of extremely inferior scores)

   c.   Mode

      —   an easily located measure of central tendency

3.   Measures of variability

In addition to measures of central tendency, it is desirable to have a measure of how the data are dispersed in either direction from the center of a distribution of scores

   a.   Range

      —   most easily calculated measure of variability
      —   obtained by subtracting the lowest score value from the highest

b. Variance

— reflects distance of the individual scores from the mean
— calculation

$$\text{variance} = \frac{\text{sum of } x^2}{n},$$

where the sum of x^2 equals the sum of squared deviations from the mean, and n = the number of cases in the distribution

c. Standard deviation

— consists of the square root of the variance
— is used to describe variability when the mean is used to describe central tendency
— while the mean is an average of the scores of a set, the standard deviation is a sort of average of how distant the individual scores in a distribution are removed from the mean itself

E. Inferential statistics

1. More complex than descriptive methods and in most instances, make use of descriptive statistics (e.g., mean and standard deviation)
2. Describe data in hand (e.g., from the sample)

a. Test for differences, as in differences between means of two groups (t test)
b. Test for relationships between variables (correlation)
c. Make predictions regarding a subject's performance on one variable, given the performance on another (regression)
d. Test for significant differences between means of two or more groups (analysis of variance)

3. Allow one to draw inferences from sample data that have wider generalizability

F. It is crucial to accept as tenable those hypotheses that are true and reject those that are false

1. The null hypothesis

a. A commonly used method of stating hypotheses in research

— postulates that there is no (null) relationship between the variables under study

        b.   The research hypothesis

            — a positive statement of the null hypothesis

   2.   Acceptance or rejection of hypotheses is based on

        a.   Statistical significance
        b.   Power
        c.   Effect size, and
        d.   Sample size

Note: An explanation of the testing of a hypothesis, with an exemplar study, may be found in Appendix D (pp.176–182). The explanation includes the concepts of statistical significance, error, directionality, and power.

II. DATA ANALYSIS AND INTERPRETATION (QUALITATIVE)

  A.   Aim: Analysis is the investigator's attempt to discover and abstract meaning. It is both creative and interactive, requiring much time, critical thinking, and emotional and conceptual energy.

  B.   Purposes

     1.   To explore and describe

        a.   Gain understanding and insight about a particular phenomenon or group of individuals

     2.   To discover and explain

        a.   Search the data to discover underlying themes, core patterns, and concepts that become the basis for inferences, interpretations and generating hypothetical statements about the meaning of the phenomenon
        b.   Analysis can be furthered to construct an explanatory scheme, model, or substantive grounded theory

     3.   Extend an existing theory to a grand or formal theory or to other contexts or other conditions

  C.   Analytic approaches

     1.   There are numerous approaches to analyzing qualitative data. Tesch (1990) identifies approximately 26 approaches to qualitative research, each having a somewhat different approach to analysis (Mariano, 1995).

      Exs. Analytic induction, content/textual analysis, thematic analysis, matrix analysis, constant comparison, phenomenological analysis, quasi-judicial analysis, discourse analysis, and narrative analysis

2. Categorical/analytic schemes or concepts can be developed directly from the data, built upon the researcher's prior research, or borrowed from the existing literature to organize and classify the data.
3. Within one approach, there may be various methods of analysis (e.g., Phenomenology: Van Manen, Giorgi, Colazzi, Van Kaam).
4. There are guidelines for data analysis, however, because each qualitative inquiry is distinctive, the analytical methods used will be unique, depending on the skills, insights, analytic abilities, and style of the investigator.

D. Elements of qualitative analysis

1. Data analysis and data collection occur concurrently, informing one another. The researcher analyzes data that have been collected and in light of that analysis, collects additional data until saturation or redundancy is reached, that is, until no new information is forthcoming from additional participants or sources. It is a cyclical, integrative, and interative process. While the researcher examines the themes and develops preliminary hypotheses throughout the progression of the study it is during the post-fieldwork stage of the research that most of the analysis and interpretation of data take place.
2. The investigator becomes immersed in and dwells with the data.
3. The researcher divides the data into smaller units for analysis (e.g., coding and categorizing), reflects on what these clusters mean, and then reintegrates them into a conceptual whole, the result being a higher-order synthesis.
4. Interpretation is required, making inferences, assigning meanings, speculating, abstracting understandings, offering explications, and dealing with disconfirming evidence, differences in data, rival hypotheses, and alternative explanations—all to test the feasibility of an interpretation
5. There is a balance between the interpretations made and the data/evidence that serves as the support for the interpretations. Conclusions are directly grounded in description, quotations, or documentary evidence.

E. Processes of qualitative analysis

1. Reflection in analysis is both personal and data oriented

    a. Personal reflection

        — feelings, assumptions, preconceived ideas, reactions, values explored and dealt with as necessary so that analysis is not merely a projection of what the researcher believes, thinks, or feels

       b.   Data-oriented reflection

         — the researcher interrogates, contemplates, dialogues with, and critically appraises the data to develop clarity of meaning and to advance the descriptive evidence to a more abstract and conceptual level

  2.   Comparison is used in disclosing conceptual similarities and differences, generating themes, and patterns, contrasting themes and patterns across individual cases/sites

  3.   Creativity is used in making sense of the data

       a.   Use of metaphor, analogy, imagery, insight

  4.   Theoretical sensitivity provides meaning and understanding

       a.   Achieved by:

         — continual verification of interpretations, hunches, and hypotheses with the actual data
         — maintenance of a skeptical stance
         — familiarity with the literature
         — adherence to sound research practices

 F.   Description of the process of data analysis

  1.   State exactly what will be done in the study

       a.   Depending on the method of analysis, will there be coding, categorizing, use of matrices, constant comparison, memoing, sorting, use of the literature, etc.?

  2.   State how the framework (if one was used) will inform the analysis of the study

  3.   Describe the use of the computer software packages for data management

III. COMPUTER SOFTWARE PACKAGES FOR QUALITATIVE DATA ANALYSIS

 A.   There is a wide variety of software tools now available to support many different approaches to qualitative data analysis

 B.   Consider type of analysis, structure of data, ease-of-use, and cost of the software

 C.   Qualitative data analysis software does not do the analysis—the researcher does. QDA software provides techniques and tools that assist the researcher in the analysis and "meaning making" process. QDA software is not a substitute for learning data analysis methods (Weitzman, 2000, p. 805)

D. Uses of QDA Software (Weitzman, p. 805), such as NUD*IST (www.qsr.com.au), HyperResearch (www.researchware.com), and Ethnograph (www.QualisResearch.com)

1. Writing field notes and memos
2. Editing
3. Coding
4. Storage
5. Search and retrieval of text and codes
6. Data "linking"
7. Content analysis using frequencies, sequences, or location of words/phrases
8. Data display
9. Graphic mapping
10. Report writing

IV. CRITERIA FOR QUALITY AND RIGOR IN QUALITATIVE RESEARCH

Measures need to be identified to ensure trustworthiness of the inquiry.

A. Credibility—assurance of plausible interpretations and conclusions

1. Prolonged engagement in the field or setting
2. Triangulation of data sources (e.g., use of a variety of sources)
3. Ongoing peer review
4. Negative case analysis (e.g., search and account for disconfirming data)
5. Member checking (e.g., having the participants review and confirm the researcher's interpretations and conclusions)

B. Transferability—permits someone else to decide if the findings of the inquiry are applicable in another setting

1. Provision of a detailed data base and "thick" description
2. The concept of applicability (applying results of a study to another population when the sample is very similar).
3. Transferability (the findings of the research hold up in other settings/situations that can be transferable to other contexts).
4. Fittingness (when findings fit into contexts different from the research situation and others find the findings meaningful and applicable to their own experiences) are used in qualitative research.

C. Dependability—determination of the reliability of the findings and interpretations that enables someone else to logically follow the process and procedures of the inquiry

1. Use of an auditor to inspect the inquiry process and the records relating to the inquiry in order to judge its authenticity

D. Confirmability—affirmation that the findings, conclusions, and recommendations are supported by or grounded in the data and that there is concordance between the researcher's interpretations and the actual evidence

   1. Use of an audit procedure
   2. Use of a reflexive journal

E. Evaluative qualities of qualitative inquiry (Mariano, 1995)

   1. Verity—Does the work ring true and is it intellectually honest and authentic?
   2. Integrity—Is the work structurally sound and is the research rationale logical and appropriate?
   3. Rigor—Is there depth of intellect rather than simplistic, superficial reasoning?
   4. Utility—Is the work useful, professionally relevant, and does it make a contribution?
   5. Vitality—Is the work meaningful, providing a sense of vibrancy and discovery, and do the metaphors and images communicate forcefully?
   6. Aesthetics—Is the work enriching, and does it touch the spirit and give others insight into some universal part of themselves?

F. Other evaluative criteria

   1. Descriptive vividness
   2. Methodological congruence (consisting of precision in documentation and procedure and strict adherence to ethics and auditability)
   3. Analytical preciseness
   4. Theoretical connectedness
   5. Heuristic relevance (which consists of intuitive recognition, relationship to existing knowledge, and applicability) (Burns, 1989).

G. Ethics

   1. Ethical issues emerge in every phase of the qualitative research process and throughout every step of the methodology
   2. Confidentiality must be assured as participants may be sharing sensitive topics and intimate details of their lives
   3. Informed consent must be secured and needs to be renegotiated over time
   4. Issues that may arise: secrets, observation of unethical or illegal activity, expectations placed on the researcher, the researcher as researcher versus "therapeutic agent" must be considered.
   5. Qualitative inquiry necessitates a continuous exploration of one's own values and ethical orientation (Mariano, 1995)

10

Product of the Inquiry:
The Research Report

I. ELEMENTS OF QUANTITATIVE RESEARCH REPORTS

    A. The abstract

        Consists of a short description of the study containing specific information

        — the research questions
        — the methods
        — the findings

    B. The introduction

        — follows the abstract
        — names the main variables or constructs of interest
        — provides the context of the research question
        — states the purpose of the study, what the researcher did, and what the researcher discovered

    C. The review of literature

        — provides current knowledge pertaining to the study problem with a brief critique
        — explains the theoretical framework
        — states the need for and significance of the study

    D. The method

    The main purpose of the Methods section is to explain the major methodological aspects of the study and why they were selected. The following aspects are usually described:

— the subjects
— the research design
— the instruments and data collection
— the study procedures

E. The results

The results of the data analyses are presented as research findings. In general, the name and value of statistical tests are presented with their statistical significance.

F. Discussion

Conclusions are drawn in the Discussion section and include:

— an interpretation of the results
— implications
— limitations of the study

II. QUALITATIVE RESEARCH REPORTS

The Research Report is a co-creation of the participant's(s') perspective of their experience and the researcher's interpretation of that experience.

A. Types of reports

1. Case report of one person, event, or institution presenting a single picture of a phenomenon in its entirety or in various stages over time
2. Narrative composite report portraying findings pertaining to a group versus one individual
3. Critical incidents
4. A grounded theory
5. A cultural ethnography
6. A phenomenological description
7. A historical narrative

B. Elements of the report

1. Problem or question
2. Detailed summary of the context/setting
3. Sample size and number of settings
4. Time and length of the inquiry
5. Researcher–participant relationship
6. Thorough representation of transactions and processes relevant to the inquiry
7. Detailed articulation of the methodology, including data gathering techniques, analytical procedures, investigator assumptions and biases, and procedures taken to ensure the rigor of the study

8. Comprehensive discussion of the results of the inquiry, interpretations a supported with substantive evidence and examples from the data, findings compared and contrasted with existing literature, and theoretical perspectives on the phenomenon

9. Implications of the study

11

Guide to Critique of Quantitative Research with Examples and Practice Studies

These are questions to consider when critiquing quantitative research. Sample critiques of two "practice" research articles are provided.

A.   The Problem

1.   In the introduction to the problem, what is the general problem of interest in the study?
2.   Does the investigator narrow the problem area to a specific problem? If so, what is the sentence that most clearly approximates a problem statement? Evaluate the statement.
3.   Does the investigator indicate the need for the study?

B.   Hypotheses or Questions

1.   If the study includes hypotheses, what are they? If the study does not include hypotheses, does the author indicate what questions the study is designed to answer? Evaluate each hypothesis or question.

C.   Variables

1.   What are the important variables in the study? Which are the independent and which are the dependent variables?

D.   Definitions

1.   Were the important variables defined operationally and conceptually? Evaluate the definitions.

E. Review of the Literature and Conceptual Framework

1. Does the investigator present a theoretical framework or a conceptual model from nursing or a related area? If so, what is it?
2. Can propositions be identified from the review of literature? Does the review indicate adequately what is known about the problem and variables of interest?

F. Method of Study

1. Research Approach

   a. What kind of research design was used?
   b. Is it appropriate for testing the hypotheses?
   c. Does the design permit control of extraneous variables? Which ones and in what way?

2. Sampling

   a. What were the actual size (n) and characteristics of the sample?
   b. Were the criteria for sample selection indicated?
   c. What was the method of sample selection? Was it the most appropriate procedure, given the circumstances?

G. Instruments

1. What instruments were used for measurement of the variables?
2. Was the reliability of each instrument previously established? Did the investigator calculate the reliability? Were the levels adequate?
3. Was the validity of each instrument formerly established? Were the levels adequate?

H. Ethics

1. If living subjects were used in the study, did the author indicate how their rights and safety were protected? If so, were the procedures adequate?

I. Analysis of Data and Presentation of Results

1. Were the data presented in relation to each hypothesis? If not, which hypothesis(es), or questions, were omitted?
2. Was a summary of all the data presented? If not, what data were collected but not presented? Was a satisfactory explanation of the omission presented?
3. Were tables included? If so, was the information presented in the tables also discussed in the text? Do the tables serve to clarify or enhance the data presentation?
4. Statistical analyses:

a.   What kinds of data were collected? (nominal, ordinal, interval, ratio?)
b.   Was a descriptive analysis of the data provided?
c.   What methods of data analyses were used? What tests of significance were used?
d.   Were the analyses appropriate to the level of data collected?

J.   Interpretations and Conclusions

1.   Are there statistically significant relationships supported in the study? If so, what are the relationships and are they interpreted?
2.   If there are contradictions between the findings and previous research, are they discussed adequately?
3.   Does the investigator relate the findings and interpretations to the framework, explaining which findings corroborate or contradict it?
4.   Do the conclusions follow logically from the results?
5.   Do the conclusions reflect all the results, both those that support the conceptual framework and those that do not?
6.   Does the investigator relate the findings to nursing practice? To education? To administration? Are indications for further research presented?

EXEMPLAR STUDY 1 WITH CRITIQUE

Youngblut, J. M., Brooten, D., Singer, L. T., Standing, T., Lee, H., & Rodgers, W. L. (2001). Effects of maternal employment and prematurity on child outcomes in single parent families. *Nursing Research 50*(6), 346–355.

A. The Problem

1. For the first time in United States' history, employment rates for single mothers have surpassed those for married mothers, due in large part to welfare reform. In 1997, 63.6% of married mothers and 65.1% of single mothers with children under 6 years of age were employed (US Bureau of the Census, 1998). Concerns about the well-being of children with employed mothers are longstanding. These concerns are of greater import for children of single mothers who have fewer resources and children at developmental risk. Premature birth, which occurs more frequently for poor single women (National Center for Health Statistics, 1995), represents a significant source of developmental risk, and a growing number of infants born prematurely survive.

2.

   a. Describe the main and interaction effects of maternal employment (employed vs. not employed) and gestational status (preterm vs. full-term) on the child's intellectual functioning and behavior;

   b. Explore the relationships between maternal employment (number of hours employed, employment history since the child's birth, and discrepancy between mothers' actual and desired employment) and the cognitive and behavioral performance of preterm and full-term preschool children; and

   c. Examine whether these relationships remained after controlling for family system and individual (mother and child) factors.

3. There is considerable research reporting the effects of maternal employment on preschool children and limited research on these effects for preschool children with developmental risk, especially for preterm children in single-parent families, where the developmental risk is greater (Singer, Yamashita, Lilien, Collin, & Baley, 1997). In view of changes in the welfare system mandating employment of poor single women, studies on the effects of maternal employment on preterm children are especially important and timely, providing data on which to base public policy and advocate effectively for these children.

   Although none of the "aims" (p. 85) were in question form, the other criteria for a research problem were met:

   #1 meets criteria for a descriptive, exploratory design;
   #2 meets criteria; and
   #3 meets criteria

B. Hypotheses or Questions

No hypothesis

C.   Variables

X_1 mother's employment

(a)   current employment status
(b)   number of hours per week
(c)   employment history since child's birth
(d)   discrepancy between actual and desired employment

X_2 child's gestational status (preterm versus full-term birth)
Y_1 cognitive performance
Y_2 behavioral performance

D.   Definitions (most operational and conceptual definitions are adequate)

1.   *Child Cognitive Function* (*Kaufman Assessment Battery for Children* [KABC] (operational)
Child's knowledge of facts, language, concepts, and school-related skills (conceptual)

Two scales

achievement—knowledge of facts, language concepts, and school-related skills
mental processes—a composite index, combining sequential and simultaneous processing subscales to yield a global estimate of intellectual functioning

(a)   discussion of construct validity (p. 86) inadequate
(b)   reliability

— internal consistency reliabilities (p. 86) adequate (.77–.82 for subscales; .86–.89 for total test)
— test-retest reliabilities adequate (.83–.88)
— interrater reliability assessed monthly *in current study* (83–100%) with retraining when in a given month fell below 90%

Raw scores were standardized by age of the child *in this study.*

2.   *The Peabody Picture Vocabulary Test-Revised* [PPVT-R] (operational)
Receptive vocabulary as an indicator of verbal intelligence (conceptual)

(a)   discussion of construct validity (p. 86) inadequate
(b)   reliability

> — test-retest reliability adequate (.76–.79)
> — internal consistency (pp. 86–87) adequate (.73–.84)
> — interrater reliability assessed monthly *in the current study* adequate (95–100%)

3. *The Child Behavior Checklist* [CBCL] (Achenbach) (operational)
   Conceptual:

   Two scales

   > internalizing—frequency of withdrawn behavior, anxious or depressed behavior, and somatic complaints
   > externalizing—frequency of aggressive and delinquent behaviors (mothers rated their children on each of 118 behaviors on a 3-point scale; after summing the ratings, raw scores were normed according to the child's age and sex)

   (a) some discussion of construct validity (p. 87) studied by author ($r = .52–.88$ with another scale)—may be inadequate
   (b) reliability

   > — test-retest reliabilities (.84–.95) adequate
   > — internal consistency reliability (.90 for internalizing subscale and .93 for externalizing subscale) adequate
   > — coefficient alpha *in this study* adequate (.83 and .91 for internalizing and externalizing subscales, respectively)

4. Employment

4a. Current employment

   Operational:

   > — employed or not employed as determined in interview (number of hours per week)

   Conceptual:

   > — none

4b. Employment history

   Background:

   Operational:

   > — *Life History Calendar* [LHC] (Freedman et al.)

Conceptual:

 — detailed descriptions of employment pattern since the study child's birth
 — when employment was started after child's birth, jobs held, months started and stopped each job, and number of hours employed per week in each job

(a) discussion of validity, based on work of Freedman et al. lends some support

Note: Authors then report modification of the LHC *for the present study* to consist of five segments (years), each with 12 blocks (months). "Recording of major life events began with the month and year of the study child's birth." Authors then added two employment variables "using LHC data": (1) proportion of the child's life the mother was employed, and (2) whether the mother was employed during the child's first year of life (yes/no)

(a) validity not adequate (no discussion)
(b) reliability not adequate (no discussion)

4c. Discrepancy between actual and desired employment

Operational:

 — computed discrepancy score between actual and desired numbers of hours per week

Conceptual:

 — none

5. Mother–Child Relationship

Parenting Stress Index [PSI] (author not clear)

One subscale: *Attachment Subscale* (operational)

Conceptual:

 — levels of strain

  (a) discussion of construct validity not adequate
  (b) discussion of internal consistency (.75), based on Abidin (1990) for the attachment subscale adequate
  (c) internal consistency *in the present study* not adequate (.66)

E.   **Review of the Literature and Conceptual Framework**

   1.   *Family Systems Theory*

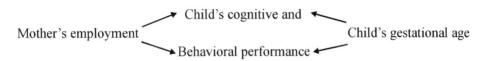

   2.   Propositions

      X_1 (a)   current employment status

             among preterm toddlers:
             employment → ↓ cognitive development
             (as compared to preterm toddlers with nonemployed mothers) (Cohen, 1978)

             among black male children in first four years of life:
             employment → ↑ vocabulary (Greenstein et al., 1995)

             among black elementary school children:
             employment → ↑ reading and achievement (Milne et al., 1986) (as compared to white)

             among girls with single mothers:
             employed full-time → ↑ academic achievement
             (as compared to girls with nonemployed single mothers) (Alessandri, 1992)

             among children of divorced mothers:
             employment → no negative effect on behavior (Kurtz & Derevensky, 1994) or academic achievement (Kinard & Reinherz, 1986)

      X_1 (b)   employment history

             among children in first or second year of life:
             employment →   ↓   adjustment
                        ↓   compliance (Belsky & Eggebeen, 1991)
                        ↓   vocabulary (Baydar & Brooks-Gunn, 1991; Desai et al., 1989)
             (findings for Desai et al. were true for sons in higher income families, in contrast to daughters in higher income families, who had higher receptive vocabulary)

             among children in first year or two of life in low income families:

employment → no negative effect on receptive vocabulary in one study (Desai et al., 1989), but

employment → ↑ receptive vocabulary (Vandall & Ramanan, 1992)

X_1 (c) number of hours per week

among preschool children:
stability of employment since birth → ↓ behavior problems (Greenstein) → positive effects (Moorhouse, 1991)

among 4-year-old children:
continuous or intermittent employment → no effect on receptive vocabulary (Desai)

X_1 (d) discrepancy between actual and desired employment

among school age children:
discrepancy → ↑ behavior problems (Barling et al., 1988)
and among kindergarten children (Auerbach et al., 1992)

at 9 and 12 months:
greater choice in whether to be employed → ↑ motor development
(Youngblut et al., 1993)

Critique

Weaknesses

— prematurity status often not reported
— statistical findings not reported; thus, cannot assess axiomatic status
— child sample broad in age range
— includes mothers who may be part of two-parent families
— theoretical frameworks not indicated
— includes other variables not initially cited (i.e., mother–child relationship, with some citations of studies)

Strengths

— *does* acknowledge that findings are mixed
— an excellent synthesis (summary) of the review of literature was presented (p. 85, paragraph preceding the aims)
— the propositions tend to support the theoretical framework but due to lack of strength and definitiveness of the studies and propositions, a clear judgment is difficult

F. Method of Study

1. Research Approach

(a) A descriptive exploratory design

(b) No hypotheses were posed; the design is appropriate for addressing the research questions (aims)

(c) There was some control over extraneous variables by means of (1) adjusting scores to be age appropriate, (2) holding some variables constant, (3) controlling for some family and individual (mother and child) factors (i.e., mother's education, total family income, number of children in the family, proportion of the child's life in a single-parent family, and attachment strains; see p. 88)

(d) Other extraneous sources of variance in outcomes that required more attention include (1) inadequate specificity in information on validity and reliability, most of which were previously established by other authors, (2) such variables as context of activity while the mother was at work (not discussed), (3) description of caretaker(s) etc.

2. Sampling

(a) The sample consisted of 121 female-headed single-parent families, half ($n = 60$) with preterm preschoolers (3, 4, or 5 years old) and half ($n = 61$) with full-term preschoolers (3, 4, or 5 years old)

(b) Inclusion criteria for the preterm children were: born prior to 36 weeks gestation, appropriate birthweight for gestational age, and hospitalized for at least 4 days in a level III NICU at birth. Inclusion criteria for the full-term children were: birth between 38 and 42 weeks gestation, discharged home with the mother after birth, and without preterm siblings who were born within 10 years of the study child's birth. For both groups, the child had to have the ability to progress intellectually. This was determined by asking mothers if they had been told their child had more than a 2-year developmental delay. None of the families were excluded on this basis.

Families were eligible to participate if the mother was not currently married and had not lived with a man serving in the father role for ≥ 6 months prior to recruitment.—criteria were comprehensive but not consistently given in cited studies

(c) Families with preterm preschoolers were identified from the admission records of three Level III Neonatal Intensive Care Units (NICUs) in the Midwest; families with full-term preschoolers were identified from birth records of newborn nurseries in two of these hospitals. A systematic random sample of families with full-term infants and all families with preterm infants born between 1988 and 1993 were sent a letter briefly describing the study; 71% of the eligible families agreed to participate.—method was appropriate given the circumstances

G. Instruments

See above

H. Ethics

— ethics were addressed (see p. 87, procedure) but informed consent for participating mothers was not addressed

I. Analysis of Data and Presentation of Results

(1) The findings were presented in relation to each of the aims.
(2) A summary of all data was presented.
(3) Tables were included and enhanced the text.
(4) Statistical analyses

(a) Nominal (i.e., yes/no) and interval data were collected
(b) Descriptive statistics were presented (i.e., sample characteristics [Table 1] and child cognitive and behavioral measures for gestational status by employment status [Table 2])

Aim 1
(c) ANOVA and MANOVA were used (see Table 2 and text). The F test of statistical significance was presented in the table. The analyses were appropriate to the interval data that were collected (see pp. 87–88 for results and detailed descriptions).

Aim 2
(c) Correlations were used to address Aim 2 (see Table 3 and text). P values of $< .05$ were used to indicate statistical significance (see p. 88 for results).

Aim 3
(c) Correlations and multiple regression analyses were used to examine Aim 3, appropriate for the level of data (interval and dichotomized or nominal (i.e., employed versus nonemployed); see pp. 88 and 90 for detailed findings).

J. Interpretations and Conclusions

At this point the student should be able to provide a comprehensive evaluation of the authors' interpretations and conclusions. SO—what do you think?

Effects of Maternal Employment and Prematurity on Child Outcomes in Single Parent Families

JoAnne M. Youngblut ▼ Dorothy Brooten ▼ Lynn T. Singer ▼ Theresa Standing ▼ Haejung Lee ▼ Willard L. Rodgers

▶ **Background:** Effects of maternal employment for preschool children vary based on specific characteristics of the mother's employment, the family's economic status, and the mother's attitudes about employment. However, there is limited research on a growing group of children at developmental risk—those born prematurely and living in a single-parent family.

▶ **Objective:** To examine the effects of maternal employment and prematurity on child cognition and behavior in single-parent families.

▶ **Methods:** Sixty preterm and 61 full-term preschool children were recruited through NICU admission records and birth records. Data were collected with the Kaufmann Assessment Battery for Children, Peabody Picture Vocabulary Test, Child Behavior Checklist, Parenting Stress Index, and the Life History Calendar.

▶ **Results:** Greater hours employed was related to higher achievement and mental processing scores only. Less discrepancy between actual and desired employment was related to higher achievement, mental processing, and language scores and lower behavior scores. Prematurity was not related to child cognitive and behavioral performance. Only the relationship between discrepancy and language remained after statistical control.

▶ **Conclusions:** The concerns about negative effects of maternal employment on young children may be overstated, especially in low-income, single-mother families. These findings are especially important in the context of welfare reform.

▶ **Key Words:** maternal employment • prematurity • single-parent families

being of children with employed mothers are longstanding. These concerns are of greater import for children of single mothers who have fewer resources and children at developmental risk. Premature birth, which occurs more frequently for poor single women (National Center for Health Statistics, 1995), represents a significant source of developmental risk, and a growing number of infants born prematurely survive. The purpose of this study was to examine the effects of the mother's employment (current employment status and number of hours employed per week, employment history since the child's birth, and discrepancy between actual and desired employment) and the child's gestational status (preterm versus full-term birth) on cognitive and behavioral performance of preschool children in a sample of female-headed, single-parent families.

There is considerable research reporting the effects of maternal employment on preschool children and limited research on these effects for preschool children with developmental risk, especially for preterm children in single-parent families, where the developmental risk is greater (Singer, Yamashita, Lilien, Collin, & Baley, 1997). In view of changes in the welfare system mandating employment of poor single women, studies on the effects of maternal employment on preterm children are especially important and timely, providing data on which to base public policy and advocate effectively for these children.

JoAnne M. Youngblut, PhD, RN, FAAN, is Professor, School of Nursing, Florida International University, Miami, and Partner, the Research A-Team, LLC.

Dorothy Brooten, PhD, RN, FAAN, is Professor, School of Nursing, Florida International University, Miami, and Partner, the Research A-Team, LLC.

Lynn T. Singer, PhD, is Associate Provost and Professor, School of Medicine, Case Western Reserve University, Cleveland, Ohio.

Theresa Standing, PhD, RN, is Director of the Doctor of Nursing Program, and Assistant Professor, Frances Payne Bolton School of Nursing, Case Western Reserve University, Cleveland, Ohio.

Haejung Lee, PhD, is Assistant Professor, Nursing Department, School of Medicine, Pusan National University, Pusan, Korea.

Willard L. Rodgers, PhD, is Senior Research Scientist, Institute for Social Research, University of Michigan, Ann Arbor, Michigan.

For the first time in United States' history, employment rates for single mothers have surpassed those for married mothers, due in large part to welfare reform. In 1997, 63.6% of married mothers and 65.1% of single mothers with children under 6 years of age were employed (US Bureau of the Census, 1998). Concerns about the well-

The organizing framework for this study is family systems theory (Bronfenbrenner, 1986; 1988). The theory posits that factors affecting one family member will have an effect on other family members, subsystems within the family (such as the parent-child dyad), and the family system as a whole. In this study, mother's employment and child gestational status are the family member factors expected to affect the child's cognitive and behavioral performance.

In the few studies on the effects of maternal employment on preterm children, findings are mixed. In an early study, preterm toddlers with employed mothers scored lower on tests of cognitive development than preterm toddlers of nonemployed mothers, controlling for birthweight and number of parents in the home (Cohen, 1978). In subsequent research with preterm infants in two-parent families, more hours employed per week was related to higher motor development scores for preterm infants at 3 months of age (Youngblut, Loveland-Cherry, & Horan, 1991), but was not related to mental and motor development at 9, 12, or 18 months (Youngblut, Loveland-Cherry, & Horan, 1993; 1994). Greenstein (1995), reporting on a large national sample which included 40% single-mother families and 8% preterm children, found no effect of prematurity or mother's current marital status on receptive vocabulary scores for preschool children. The only effect of maternal employment in that sample was for Black male children who scored higher on vocabulary when their mothers were employed during their first 4 years of life.

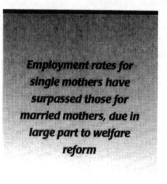

Employment rates for single mothers have surpassed those for married mothers, due in large part to welfare reform

▼▼▼

Maternal employment in single-parent families has either positive effects or no effects for children. Milne, Myers, Rosenthal, and Ginsburg (1986) found higher reading and math achievement scores for Black, but not White, elementary school children with employed single mothers. Alessandri (1992) found that girls with single mothers who were employed full-time had higher academic achievement than girls with nonemployed single mothers. However, Hall, Gurley, Sachs, and Kryscio (1991) found no differences between employed and nonemployed low-income single mothers in their perceptions of their preschool child's behavior. These findings remained after statistically controlling for income, race, social desirability, level of stress, coping, and parenting attitudes. Maternal employment had no negative effects on behavior (Kurtz & Derevensky, 1994; Pett, Vaughan-Cole, & Wampold, 1994) or academic achievement (Kinard & Reinherz, 1986) for children of divorced mothers.

Studies of the effects of maternal employment on the child have investigated not only employment status and number of hours worked, but also mother's employment history and employment preference. Maternal employment during the child's first or second year of life has been reported to have a negative effect on preschool children's adjustment and compliance (Belsky & Eggebeen, 1991)

and receptive vocabulary (Baydar & Brooks-Gunn, 1991; Desai, Chase-Lansdale, & Michael, 1989). However, the findings of Desai and colleagues held only for sons in higher income families; in contrast, daughters in higher income families had higher receptive vocabulary. In low-income families, maternal employment in the first year or two of life had no effect on children's receptive vocabulary in one study (Desai et al., 1989) but had positive effects for children in another (Vandall & Ramanan, 1992).

Research on the effects of the stability of the mothers' employment on children also has reported mixed results. Greenstein (1993) found that preschool children whose mothers were continuously employed since their birth had fewer behavior problems. In families where the mother was either not employed or employed intermittently, quality of the home environment was an important factor in predicting child behavior. Moorehouse (1991) also found positive effects for stability in employment pattern. In that study, 6-year-old children whose mothers changed their employment during the previous 3 years scored significantly lower on teachers' ratings of their cognitive and social competence than children whose mothers were continuously employed. In another study, Desai et al. (1989) found no effect of continuous or intermittent maternal employment on 4-year-old children's receptive vocabulary.

Discrepancy between actual and desired employment often is found to have negative effects for children, especially when employed and nonemployed mothers are both included in the study. Discrepancy between actual and desired employment has been associated with behavior problems for school-age (Barling, Fullagar, & Marchl-Dingle, 1988) and kindergarten children (Auerbach, Lerner, Barasch, & Palti, 1992). Mothers' greater choice in whether to be employed was related to higher motor development scores at 9 and 12 months (Youngblut et al., 1993) and higher mental development scores at 18 months (Youngblut et al., 1994) for preterm infants in two-parent families.

However, for employed mothers, the discrepancy between actual and desired employment may have no effect for children's behavior and development. Indeed, Youngblut, Singer, Madigan, Swegart, and Rodgers (1998) found that discrepancy was not related to parenting strains for employed single mothers, but was associated with greater parenting strains for nonemployed single mothers. In a sample of poor, Black, single, employed mothers of preschoolers, Jackson (1993) found that employment preference was not related to mothers' perceptions of their preschool children's behavior. However, mothers who preferred to be employed expressed greater life satisfaction and less role strain than those who preferred not to be employed. MacEwen and Barling (1991) also found no relationship between employed married mothers' satisfaction with their employee roles and their children's behavior. Thus, as in an early study by Farel (1980), discrepancy between the mother's actual and desired employment may be particularly important for families where the mother is not employed.

In summary, research findings to date on the effects of maternal employment on the development of children in single-parent families show positive effects or no effect. Studies examining maternal employment begun in the first year or two of life demonstrate negative effects on preschool children's receptive vocabulary scores, adjustment, and compliance; however, family income has been found to mediate these effects. For employed mothers who wish to work, research has demonstrated greater life satisfaction and less parenting role strain. Research on employed mothers not wanting to work has shown no reported negative effects on child behavior or development. Nonemployed mothers wishing to work report parenting strain. There are few studies of the effects of maternal employment on a growing group of children at developmental risk, those born prematurely. Research is even more limited in this group born to single mothers, who deliver a greater portion of these newborns. The aims of this research were to:

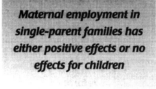

Maternal employment in single-parent families has either positive effects or no effects for children

1. Describe the main and interaction effects of maternal employment (employed vs. not employed) and gestational status (preterm vs. full-term) on the child's intellectual functioning and behavior;
2. Explore the relationships between maternal employment (number of hours employed, employment history since the child's birth, and discrepancy between mothers' actual and desired employment) and the cognitive and behavioral performance of preterm and full-term preschool children; and
3. Examine whether these relationships remained after controlling for family system and individual (mother and child) factors. These aims are part of a larger study of maternal employment effects for families with preterm and full-term preschool children (Youngblut & Brooten, 2000; Youngblut, Singer, Madigan, Swegart, & Rodgers, 1997; Youngblut et al., 1998)

Method

Sample: The sample consisted of 121 female-headed single-parent families, half ($n = 60$) with preterm preschoolers (3, 4, or 5 years old) and half ($n = 61$) with full-term preschoolers (3, 4, or 5 years old) Families with preterm preschoolers were identified from the admission records of three Level III Neonatal Intensive Care Units (NICUs) in the Midwest; families with full-term preschoolers were identified from birth records of newborn nurseries in two of these hospitals. A systematic random sample of families with full-term infants and all families with preterm infants born between 1988 and 1993 were sent a letter briefly describing the study; 71% of the eligible families agreed to participate.

Inclusion criteria for the preterm children were: born prior to 36 weeks gestation, appropriate birthweight for gestational age, and hospitalized for at least 4 days in a level III NICU at birth. Inclusion criteria for the full-term children were: birth between 38 and 42 weeks gestation, discharged home with the mother after birth, and without preterm siblings who were born within 10 years of the study child's birth. For both groups, the child had to have the ability to progress intellectually. This was determined by asking mothers if they had been told their child had more than a 2-year developmental delay. None of the families were excluded on this basis.

Families were eligible to participate if the mother was not currently married and had not lived with a man serving in the father role for ≥6 months prior to recruitment. Five index children were being raised by a single woman other than the birth mother (1 adoptive mother, 2 grandmothers, and 2 foster mothers). In each case, the child had lived with the family for most of the child's life and the woman was performing the role of "mother" to the child. Thus, these women are referred to here as "mothers."

Most mothers were African American (66.1%), had completed high school (76.9%), had never been married (70.2%), and had sole custody of the study child (92.5%). The sample was comprised of primarily low-income families; 61.1% received public assistance, 66.1% received less than $3,000 annually through the mother's employment, and 93.3% had total family incomes under $20,000 per year. Only 17.4% of the mothers received child support from the child's father. Table 1 compares family characteristics for the preterm and full-term groups. Families in the two groups did not differ significantly on any of the demographic variables, except for the child's birthweight and gestational age.

About half of the children in the sample were male (52.9%) and first-born (44.6%). Birthweight ranged from 470 to 2,460 grams for the preterm group; 12 (20%) had birth weights less than 1,000 grams, 23 (38.3%) had birth weights between 1,000 and 1,499 grams, and 25 (41.7%) had birth weights between 1,500 and 2,500 grams. Birthweight for the full-term group ranged from 2,515 to 4,965 grams. Gestational age ranged from 24 to 35 weeks for the preterm children and from 36 to 42 weeks for the full-term children. Although the bottom cutoff for gestational age at birth for full-term children was 38 weeks, 4 full-term children who were 37 weeks gestation at birth were recruited. Because these children were healthy, not hospitalized in the NICU, and discharged home with their mothers after birth, they were included in the full-term sample.

The preterm children had spent an average of 46.1 days ($SD = 33.34$, range 4 to 128 days) in the NICU at birth. One-third were discharged by 1 month of age, another third by 2 months of age. A few preterm preschoolers had experienced complications of prematurity. Thirteen experi-

TABLE I. Comparison of Families With Preterm and Full Term Preschoolers			
Characteristic	Preterm M (SD)	Full Term M (SD)	Statistic
Mother's age	29.90 (6.86)	29.20 (6.17)	$t = .58$
Proportion child's life employed	.27 (.37)	.22 (.32)	$t = .78$
Discrepancy	20.80 (12.94)	21.00 (14.59)	$t = .08$
Number of children	2.50 (1.55)	2.50 (1.34)	$t = .13$
Child's age (months)	48.70 (9.92)	48.40 (9.96)	$t = .18$
Birthweight (grams)	1444.10 (527.21)	3331.30 (514.18)	$t = 19.93^*$
Gestational age at birth (weeks)	30.50 (3.17)	39.60 (1.60)	$t = 19.98^*$
Proportion child's life single	.89 (.26)	.88 (.24)	$t = .23$
Mother's race	N (%)	N (%)	
White	16 (13%)	23 (19%)	$\chi^2 = 4.05$
Black	44 (36%)	36 (30%)	
Hispanic	0 (0%)	2 (2%)	
Mother's education			
<High school	12 (10%)	16 (13%)	$\chi^2 = 1.15$
High school grad	20 (16%)	22 (18%)	
>High school	28 (23%)	23 (19%)	
Family income			
<$20,000	51 (85%)	60 (98%)	$\chi^2 = 5.23$
$20,000–39,999	6 (10%)	1 (2%)	
≥$40,000	3 (5%)	0 (0%)	
Mother's employment status			
Employed	17 (14%)	17 (14%)	$\chi^2 = .003$
Nonemployed	43 (35%)	44 (36%)	
Child's sex			
Female	32 (26%)	25 (21%)	$\chi^2 = 1.85$
Male	28 (23%)	36 (30%)	

$^*p < .01.$

enced an intraventricular hemorrhage; 10 were Grade I, and there was one child each with Grades II, III, and IV. Two children were diagnosed with cerebral palsy and two with bronchopulmonary dysplasia.

At the time of the study, 34 (28.1%) women were employed, 27 full-time (≥30 hours per week) and 7 part-time (<30 hours per week), $M = 34.3$ hours/week ($SD = 10.23$). Women's self-reported "usual" occupations were classified as homemakers (42.2%), unskilled (7.4%), skilled or semi-skilled (19.8%), clerical or sales (14.1%), and professionals (16.5%).

Instruments: Child Cognitive Functioning: The Kaufman Assessment Battery for Children (KABC) was designed for children between 2.5 and 12.5 years old and contains two scales: achievement and mental processes. The achievement scale assesses the child's knowledge of facts, language concepts, and school-related skills. The mental processes scale is a composite index, combining sequential and simultaneous processing subscales to yield a global estimate of intellectual functioning. Items are presented to the child and his/her responses scored. Pictures and diagrams are frequently used as test materials, with few verbal responses required. As recommended, raw scores were standardized by age of the child in this study. Extensive testing supports the construct validity of the measure (Merz, 1984). Internal consistency reliabilities are reported to range from .77 to .82 for the subscales and from .86 to .89 for the total test; test-retest reliabilities range from .83 to .88 (Bracken, 1987). Interrater reliability (percent agreement), assessed monthly in the current study, ranged from 83–100% ($M = 95.8\%$). Retraining occurred when the interrater reliability in a given month fell below 90%.

The Peabody Picture Vocabulary Test-Revised: The PPVT-R (Dunn & Dunn, 1981) was used to measure receptive vocabulary as an indicator of verbal intelligence; it can be used with people from 2.5 years of age through adulthood. Children were presented with pictures and their responses scored. As recommended, raw scores were standardized by age of the respondent. Construct validity is supported through correlations with various IQ scales in previous research. For preschoolers, test-retest reliability is reported to range from .76 to .79 and internal consistency, from .73 to .84 (Bracken, 1987). Interrater reliability, assessed monthly in the current study, ranged from 95–100% ($M = 99.0\%$).

Child Behavioral Performance: The Child Behavior Checklist (CBCL; Achenbach, 1991) was used to measure children's behavior problems. The internalizing scale measures frequency of withdrawn behavior, anxious or depressed behavior, and somatic complaints; the externalizing scale measures frequency of aggressive and delinquent behaviors. Mothers rated their children on each of 118 behaviors on a 3-point scale ranging from "not true" to "often true." After summing the mothers' ratings, raw scores were normed according to the child's age and sex. The behavior problems subscales of the CBCL have been widely used with documented evidence for their construct validity. Achenbach reports moderate to strong correlations between the internalizing and externalizing subscales and similar scales of the Quay-Peterson Revised Behavior Problem Checklist ($r = .52–.88$); test-retest reliabilities of .84 to .95; and internal consistency reliability of .90 for the internalizing subscale and .93 for the externalizing subscale. In this study, coefficient alpha was .83 and .91 for internalizing and externalizing subscales, respectively.

Improvements in neonatal care have resulted in high-risk neonates surviving with less impairment

Current Employment: Current employment was classified as employed or not employed based on mothers' stated employment during interview. Mothers provided number of hours per week they currently work.

Employment History: Mothers gave detailed descriptions of their employment pattern since the study child's birth on a Life History Calendar (LHC) (Freedman, Thornton, Camburn, Alwin, & Young-DeMarco, 1988). This included when they began employment after the child's birth, the jobs they had held, the months they started and stopped each job, and the number of hours employed per week in each job. Validity and reliability of the LHC is enhanced through its use of memory cues, relating one event to other events that occurred at about the same time. When Freedman et al. compared data obtained in 1980 about the respondent's current situation with data obtained retrospectively with the LHC in 1985 ($N = 900$), agreement ranged from 72% to 92%. The LHC constructed for the current study contained five segments (years), each with 12 blocks (months). Major life events, such as residential moves, births, deaths, and hospitalizations of the study child, also were recorded to aid the mother's memory. Recording began with the month and year of the study child's birth. From the LHC data, two additional employment variables were created: the proportion of the child's life the mother was employed and whether the mother was employed during the child's first year of life (yes/no).

Discrepancy Between Actual and Desired Employment: Discrepancy between actual and desired employment was measured with a computed discrepancy score. Mothers indicated the number of hours per week they would prefer to work outside the home. Discrepancy scores were then computed by subtracting the actual number of work hours from the preferred number of work hours and taking the absolute value. Higher scores indicate greater discrepancy. Only five of the nonemployed mothers in this sample indicated they preferred not to work. Nonemployed mothers reported considerably more discrepancy than employed mothers, $M = 25.9$ ($SD = 13.13$) and $M = 9.5$ ($SD = 6.48$), respectively, $t = 8.80$, $p < .01$.

Mother-Child Relationship: Mother-child relationship was measured with the 7-item attachment subscale of the Parenting Stress Index (PSI). Mothers rated each item on a 5-point Likert scale from 1 "strongly agree" to 5 "strongly disagree." Higher scores indicate higher levels of strain. Sample items include: "It takes a long time for parents to develop close, warm feelings for their children" and "Sometimes my child does things that bother me just to be mean." Construct validity of the PSI is supported by group differences between parents of children with and without disabilities. Abidin (1990) reported internal consistency of .75 for the attachment subscale. Internal consistency in this study was .66.

Procedure: The study was approved by the appropriate Human Subjects Review committees at the university and each of the three hospitals. A trained interviewer then contacted the family to screen for inclusion criteria, answer questions, and schedule a data collection visit in the family's home. Interviewers offered to read self-complete instruments to mothers.

Results

Aim 1: Describe the main and interaction effects of maternal employment (employed vs. not employed) and gestational status (preterm vs. full-term) on the child's intellectual functioning and behavior.

Children of employed mothers scored significantly higher on achievement than children of nonemployed mothers, regardless of gestational status. In addition, employed mothers of preterm preschoolers reported significantly fewer externalizing behavior problems than other mothers (Table 2). The main and interaction effects of current maternal employment (employed vs. not employed) and child gestational status at birth (full-term or preterm) on the cognitive (KABC mental processes and achievement, PPVT-R) and behavioral measures (CBCL internalizing [withdrawn behavior, anxious or depressed behavior, and somatic complaints] and externalizing [aggressive and delinquent behaviors] behavior problems) were analyzed

TABLE 2. Descriptive Statistics for Child Cognitive and Behavioral Measures for Gestational Status by Employment Status Groups

	Groups					
	EM Preterm (n = 17) M (SD)	NEM Preterm (n = 42) M (SD)	EM Fullterm (n = 17) M (SD)	NEM Fullterm (n = 44) M (SD)	Significant Effects	F
Cognitive measures					Employment[a]	2.63*
Achievement	91.9 (13.64)	85.9 (10.63)	94.1 (11.54)	87.1 (11.10)	Employment[b]	7.85**
Mental processes	97.9 (16.98)	91.4 (14.45)	95.9 (8.85)	92.6 (14.93)	None[b]	NS
PPVT-R	80.7 (16.51)	79.0 (18.42)	87.2 (12.72)	78.3 (17.84)	None[b]	NS
Behavioral measures					Interaction[a]	3.45*
Internalizing	46.9 (9.04)	49.4 (10.80)	44.9 (8.73)	47.8 (10.17)	None[b]	NS
Externalizing	46.5 (6.43)	54.7 (11.68)	54.2 (10.14)	54.0 (10.54)	Interaction[b]	3.79*

Note. EM = employed mothers; NEM = nonemployed mothers; PPVT-R = Peabody Picture Vocabulary Test—Revised.
[a]MANOVA results.
[b]ANOVA results.
*p < .05, **p < .01.

with two-way MANOVA because of the substantial inter-correlation among the three cognitive measures, $r = .52$ to 66, and between the two behavior measures, $r = .62$. Correlations between the cognitive measures and the behavior measures were weak, $r = -.13$ to $-.20$, indicating the need for separate MANOVAs. For the cognitive measures, the interaction effect of employment and prematurity and the main effect of prematurity were not significant. However, there was a significant main effect of employment. Post-hoc univariate ANOVA showed significant group differences only on children's achievement, with children of employed mothers scoring higher than children of nonemployed mothers. Analysis of the behavioral measures revealed a significant interaction effect of employment and prematurity. Post-hoc univariate ANOVA found a significant interaction effect on externalizing behavior problems only; employed mothers of preterm preschoolers reported fewer externalizing behavior problems than other mothers.

Aim 2: Examine the relationships between maternal employment (number of hours employed, employment history since the child's birth, and discrepancy between mothers' actual and desired employment) and cognitive and behavioral performance of preterm and full-term preschool children.

Employment was significantly related to child cognitive and behavioral performance measures, before controlling for the effects of other variables (Table 3). The more hours the mother was employed per week, the higher her child's achievement and mental processes scores. Children whose mothers worked during their first year of life had higher language scores (PPVT-R). Correlations of the proportion of the child's life the mother was employed with the cognitive and behavior measures were weak and not significant. Greater discrepancy between actual and desired employment was related to lower achievement, mental processes, and language scores; and more externalizing and internal-

izing behavior problems. Prematurity was not significantly related to the cognitive and behavioral measures.

Aim 3: Examine whether these relationships remain after controlling for family system and individual (mother and child) factors.

Multiple regression analyses (Tables 4 and 5) were used to investigate the effect of mother's employment, discrepancy between actual and desired employment, and gestational status on child cognitive and behavioral performance, controlling for mother's education, total family income, number of children in the family, proportion of the child's life in a single-parent family, and attachment strains. Two correlations among the independent variables were >.60: proportion of the child's life with an employed mother with current number of hours employed ($r = .64$) and with maternal employment during the child's first year of life ($r = .66$). Maternal employment was represented with an interval level variable (number of hours employed per week) in half the regressions and with a dichotomized variable (employed/not employed) in the other half. Likewise, employment history was represented with an interval level variable (proportion of the child's life with an employed mother) in half of the regressions, and with a dichotomized variable (employed/not employed in child's first year of life) in the other half. This was done to investigate the effects of timing of maternal employment (Baydar & Brooks-Gunn, 1991; Belsky & Eggebeen, 1991; Desai et al., 1989).

Current maternal employment, employment history, and gestational status were not significantly related to child cognitive and behavioral performance. Greater discrepancy between actual and desired maternal employment was significantly related only to lower receptive language scores. Several of the control variables were significant predictors of child cognitive and behavior problem measures. Higher family income was a significant predictor of both

TABLE 3. Correlations Among Employment, Control, and Child Cognitive and Behavioral Variables

	2	3	4	5	6	7	8	9	10	11	12	13	14	15
Total Sample														
1 Mother's education	.31**	−.29**	−.17	.10	−.04	.29**	.16	.31**	−.15	.15	.11	−.03	−.08	−.21*
2 Family income		.01	−.18	.13	−.08	.43**	.20*	.26**	−.16	.24**	.17	.15	−.01	.07
3 No. children in family			.11	.01	.08	−.17	−.24**	−.33**	.12	−.35**	−.06	−.32**	−.07	.21*
4 Proportion child's life single				.02	.06	−.09	−.09	−.13	.11	−.18	−.13	−.07	−.02	.14
5 Gestational status (1 = preterm)					.02	.01	.17	.07	−.008	−.06	−.01	−.04	−.09	.08
6 Attachment strains						−.19*	−.01	−.09	.28**	−.23*	−.15	−.17	.28**	.29**
7 Hours employed per week							.44**	.64**	−.51**	.29**	.20*	.17	−.18	−.12
8 Worked in first year of life?								.66**	−.14	.13	.08	.20*	−.06	−.06
9 Proportion child's life employed									−.34**	.16	.06	.13	−.10	−.09
10 Discrepancy										−.28**	−.24**	−.27**	.27**	.20*
11 Achievement (KABC)											.66**	.66**	−.13	−.19*
12 Mental processes (KABC)												.52**	−.16	−.15
13 PPVT-R													−.13	−.15
14 Externalizing behavior														.62**
15 Internalizing behavior														—

Note. KABC = Kaufman Assessment Battery for Children; PPVT-R = Peabody Picture Vocabulary Test—Revised.
*p < .05.
**p < .01.

Independent Variables	Achievement				Mental Process				PPVT-R			
Mother's education	.03	-.01	-.01	-.03	-.01	-.01	-.01	.01	-.21*	-.21*	-.20	-.17
Total family income	.17	.25*	.24**	.19	.08	.11	.13	.11	.21*	.21*	.21*	.18
Gestational status (preterm=1, fullterm=0)	-.02	-.04	-.05	-.02	.01	-.02	-.03	.0009	-.09	-.09	-.09	-.06
Number children in family	-.33**	-.30**	-.30**	-.33**	.02	.06	.06	.02	-.31**	-.31**	-.31**	-.35**
Proportion child's life with single mother	.01	-.02	-.02	.01	-.06	-.07	-.06	-.06	.07	.07	.07	.07
Attachment strains	-.08	-.09	-.10	-.09	-.04	-.06	-.06	-.05	-.07	-.07	-.06	-.07
Discrepancy	-.20	-.20	-.20	-.22	.16	-.15	-.18	-.17	-.24*	-.24*	-.26*	-.23
Hours employed per week	.14	—	—	—	-.10	—	—	—	-.09	—	—	—
Employment (EM = 1, NEM = 0)	—	-.07	—	—	—	.01	—	—	—	.11	—	—
Proportion child's life with employed mother	—	—	-.02	—	—	—	.09	—	—	—	.16	—
Resumed employment in 1st year of life	—	—	—	.0007	—	—	—	-.04	—	—	—	.05
F	3.29**	3.81**	3.75**	3.19**	.85	1.10	1.08	.74	2.48**	2.93**	2.97**	2.49**
Adjusted R^2	.18	.20	.20	.17	.00	.01	.01	.00	.12	.15	.15	.12

TABLE 4. Multiple Regression[a] of Child Cognitive Development on Employment and Control Variables

Note. For explanation of abbreviations, see footnote to Table 2.
*p < .05.
**p < .01.
[a] all regression coefficients standardized.

higher achievement scores and higher PPVT-R scores. Higher maternal education was related to higher PPVT-R scores and fewer internalizing behavior problems. In addition, fewer children in the family was related to higher achievement and PPVT-R scores and greater externalizing behavior problems. Mother-child attachment strains were a significant predictor for behavior problems only, with greater strains related to greater externalizing and internalizing behavior problems.

Discussion

In this sample of female-headed, single-parent, primarily low-income families, more hours of maternal employment was related to better child outcomes in cognition and achievement. However, when family, child, and maternal factors were controlled, the beneficial effect of the mother's employment was no longer significant. This finding is consistent with those of other studies with low-income and/or single-parent families (Hall et al., 1991; Kinard & Reinherz, 1986; Kurtz & Derevensky, 1994; Pett et al., 1994). Thus, mothers' employment in single-parent families may result in more positive child outcomes not because of the employment itself but because of the greater financial resources and improved feelings of self-worth (Hall et al., 1991) the mothers' employment usually brings.

Less discrepancy between the mother's actual and desired employment was related to better child cognition, achievement, language, and behavioral performance. However, when other factors were controlled, only the positive effects for receptive language remained significant. Other studies also have found negative effects of discrepancy for the child (Auerbach et al., 1992; Barling et al., 1988; Youngblut et al., 1993; 1994). As others have suggested, mothers whose actual and desired employment status do not match may be depressed, with fewer emotional resources to be responsive and positive to their children (Farel, 1980; Hock & DeMeis, 1990).

Duration and timing of maternal employment contributed very little to child cognitive and behavioral performance when considered alone and after controlling for other variables. Employment during the child's first year was related to higher receptive language scores, but only when no statistical controls were applied, and proportion of the child's life with an employed mother was not related to child cognitive and behavioral performance, both with and without statistical controls. Although Belsky and Eggebeen (1991) and Baydar and Brooks-Gunn (1991) found negative effects of early employment, Vandell and Ramanan (1992) found positive effects of early maternal employment for children in low-income families. In a sample of mixed-income families, Desai et al. (1989) found that outcomes for children in low-income families were not related to either the child's age when the mother began employment or the mother's pattern of employment.

Prematurity had no effect on any of the child outcome measures in this study. This is in contrast to other studies of preterm children that have found significant cognitive delays (Hack et al., 1997) or behavior problems (Brandt et

TABLE 5. Multiple Regression[a] of Child Behavior on Employment and Control Variables

Independent Variables	Externalizing Behavior Problems			Internalizing Behavior Problems		
Mother's education	-.11	-.11	-.11	-.29**	-.29**	-.29**
Total family income	.07	.06	.07	.22*	.18	.22*
Gestational status (preterm = 1, fullterm = 0)	-.06	-.06	-.06	.08	.08	.08
Number children in family	-.20	-.22*	-.23*	.09	.07	.09
Proportion child's life with single mother	-.09	-.10	-.10	.05	.07	.05
Attachment strains	.28**	.23**	.28**	.26**	.26**	.25*
Discrepancy	.17	.21	.20	.12	.14	.13
Hours employed per week	.003	.01	—	.07	.07	—
Employment status (EM = 1, NEM = 0)	—	—	.02	—	—	—
Proportion child's life with employed mother	-.09	—	—	-.02	-.06	-.07
Resumed employment in 1st year of life	—	-.13	-.12	—	-.03	-.02
F	1.99*	2.53**	2.53**	2.65**	2.84**	2.66**
Adjusted R^2	.09	.12	.12	.14	.14	.14

*$p < .05$.
**$p < .01$.
[a]all regression coefficients standardized.

al., 1992) into the school-age years. Two aspects of our study may account for the conflicting findings. Our sample is a healthier, less impaired sample because children were recruited from birth records, not from developmental follow-up clinics. Preterm children in this sample were born later than those in the studies by Hack et al. and Brandt et al. Improvements in neonatal care, such as use of surfactant to speed lung maturity in very young preterm infants, have resulted in high-risk neonates surviving with less impairment. Indeed, neurologic impairment and respiratory risk, rather than prematurity, predicted negative outcomes in the study by Singer et al. (1997).

In addition, we considered the effects of environmental factors known to influence child outcomes. Other studies of preterm children often include both single-parent and two-parent families in their samples and do not control statistically for the differences in family structure or the effects of other family factors such as number of children in the family and family income. Although the sample was relatively homogeneous on income, both income and number of children had significant effects on child cognitive and behavioral performance in this study regardless of the child's gestational age at birth. It is also likely that the pervasive effects of poverty (Bolger, Patterson, Thompson, & Kuperschmidt, 1995) are stronger than the effects of prematurity in a low-income sample by the time the child reaches preschool age. Indeed, Singer et al. (1997) found that neurologic risk, low social class, and minority race mediated the effects of birthweight and gestational age on outcomes of very low birthweight infants at 3 years of age. Thus, our lack of effects for prematurity is probably due to a healthier, less impaired preterm sample combined with the strong effects of poverty on child cognitive and behavioral performance.

In summary, current maternal employment, employment history, and discrepancy between actual and desired employment had little to no effect on child cognitive and behavioral outcomes in this sample of preterm and full-term children in single-parent, primarily low-income families. Prematurity also was not related to child cognitive and behavioral performance. However, fewer children in the family had consistent, positive effects for the child outcomes in this study. The concerns about negative effects of maternal employment on young children may be overstated, especially in low income, female-headed single-parent families. The current welfare reform legislation mandating employment for single mothers with young children holds the potential, given current research, of having no effect or positive effects on child development. Potential effects of maternal employment in single-parent families, however, will require ongoing monitoring, particularly for groups of children at developmental risk. ▼

Accepted for publication April 10, 2001.

This study was supported by grant # R01 NR02707 from the National Institute of Nursing Research and an administrative supplement from the Office of Research on Women's Health, National Institutes of Health.

Address correspondence to: JoAnne M. Youngblut, PhD, RN, FAAN, School of Nursing, Florida International University, 3000 NE 151st Street, AC II, Room 234A, North Miami, FL 33181 (e-mail: youngblu@fin.edu).

References

Achenbach, T. M. (1991). *Manual for the Child Behavior Checklist/4-18 and 1991 Profile.* Burlington, VT: University of Vermont Department of Psychiatry.

Abidin, R. R. (1990). *Parenting stress index manual* (3rd ed.). Charlottesville, VA: Pediatric Psychology Press.

Alessandri, S. M. (1992). Effects of maternal work status in single-parent families on children's perception of self and family and school achievement. *Journal of Experimental Child Psychology, 54,* 417-433.

Auerbach, J., Lerner, Y., Barasch, M., & Palti, H. (1992). Maternal and environmental characteristics as predictors of child behavior problems and cognitive competence. *American Orthopsychiatric Association, 62,* 409-420.

Barling, J., Fullagar, C., & Marchl-Dingle, J. (1988). Employment commitment as a moderator of the maternal employment status/child behavior relationship. *Journal of Organizational Behavior, 9,* 113-122.

Baydar, N., & Brooks-Gunn, J. (1991). Effects of maternal employment and child care arrangements on preschoolers' cognitive and behavioral outcomes: Evidence from the children of the National Longitudinal Study of Youth. *Developmental Psychology, 27,* 932-945.

Belsky, J., & Eggbeen, D. (1991). Early and extensive maternal employment and young children's socioemotional development: Children of the National Longitudinal Survey of Youth. *Journal of Marriage & the Family, 53,* 1083-1110.

Bolger, K. E., Patterson, C. J., Thompson, W. W., & Kupersmidt, J. B. (1995). Psychosocial adjustment among children experiencing persistent and intermittent family economic hardship. *Child Development, 66,* 1107-1129.

Bracken, B. A. (1987). Limitations of preschool instruments and standards for minimal levels of technical adequacy. *Journal of Psychoeducational Assessment, 4,* 313-326.

Brandt, P., Magyary, D., Hammond, M., & Barnard, K. (1992). Learning and behavioral-emotional problems of children born preterm at second grade. *Journal of Pediatric Psychology, 17,* 291-311.

Bronfenbrenner, U. (1986). Ecology of the family as a context for human development. *Developmental Psychology, 22,* 723-742.

Bronfenbrenner, U. (1988). Ecological systems theory. *Annals of Child Development, 6,* 187-249.

Cohen, S. E. (1978). Maternal employment and mother-child interaction. *Merrill-Palmer Quarterly, 24,* 189-197.

Desai, S., Chase-Lansdale, P. L., & Michael, R. T. (1989). Mother or market? Effects of maternal employment on the intellectual ability of 4-year-old children. *Demography, 26,* 545-561.

Dunn, L. M., & Dunn, L. M. (1981). *Peabody Picture Vocabulary Test-Revised.* Circle Pines, MN: American Guidance Service.

Farel, A. (1980). Effects of preferred maternal roles, maternal employment, and sociodemographic status on school adjustment and competence. *Child Development, 51,* 1179-1186.

Freedman, D., Thornton, A., Camburn, D., Alwin, D., & Young-DeMarco, L. (1988). The Life History Calendar: A technique for collecting retrospective data. *Sociological Methodology, 18,* 37-68.

Greenstein, T. N. (1993). Maternal employment and child behavioral outcomes. *Journal of Family Issues, 14,* 323-354.

Greenstein, T. N. (1995). Are the "most advantaged" children truly disadvantaged by early maternal employment? *Journal of Family Issues, 16,* 149-169.

Hack, M., Breslau, N., Aram, D., Weissman, B., Klein, N., & Borawski-Clark, E. (1992). The effect of very low birth weight and social risk on neurocognitive abilities at school age. *Journal of Developmental and Behavioral Pediatrics, 13,* 412-420.

Hall, L. A., Gurley, D. N., Sachs, B., & Kryscio, R. J. (1991). Psychosocial predictors of maternal depressive symptoms, parenting attitudes, and child behavior in single-parent families. *Nursing Research, 40,* 214-220.

Hock, E., & DeMeis, D. (1990). Depression in mothers of infants: The role of maternal employment. *Developmental Psychology, 26,* 285-291.

Jackson, A. P. (1993). Black, single, working mothers in poverty: Preferences for employment, well-being, and perceptions of preschool-age children. *Social Work, 38,* 26-34.

Kinard, E. M., & Reinherz, H. (1986). Effects of marital disruption of children's school aptitude and achievement. *Journal of Marriage & the Family, 48,* 285-293.

Kurtz, L., & Derevensky, J. L. (1994). Family configuration and maternal employment: Effects on family environment and children's outcomes. *Journal of Divorce and Remarriage, 22,* 137-154.

MacEwen, K. E., & Barling, J. (1991). Effects of maternal employment experiences on children's behavior via mood, cognitive difficulties, and parenting behavior. *Journal of Marriage and the Family, 53,* 635-644.

Merz, W. R. (1984). Kaufman assessment battery for children. In D. J. Keyser & R. C. Sweetland (Eds.), *Test Critiques.* Kansas City, MO: Test Corporation of America.

Milne, A. M., Myers, D. E., Rosenthal, A. S., & Ginsburg, A. (1986). Single parents, working mothers and the educational achievement of school children. *Sociology of Education, 59,* 125-139.

Moorehouse, M. J. (1991). Linking maternal employment patterns to mother-child activities and children's school competence. *Developmental Psychology, 27,* 295-303.

National Center for Health Statistics. (1995). Health aspects of childbearing by unmarried women. *Vital and Health Statistics, 21*(53), 19-23.

Pett, M. A., Vaughan-Cole, B., & Wampold, B. E. (1994). Maternal employment and perceived stress: Their impact on children's adjustment and mother-child interaction in young divorced and married families. *Family Relations, 43,* 151-158.

Singer, L. T., Yamashita, T. S., Lilien, L., Collin, M., & Baley, J. (1997). A longitudinal study of infants with bronchopulmonary dysplasia and very low birthweight. *Pediatrics, 100,* 987-993.

U.S. Bureau of the Census. (1998). *Statistical Abstract of the United States,* 116th Ed. Washington, DC: US Government Printing Office.

Vandell, D. L., & Ramanan, J. (1992). Effects of early and recent maternal employment on children from low-income families. *Child Development, 63,* 938-949.

Youngblut, J. M., & Brooten, D. (1999). Alternate child care, history of hospitalization, and preschool child behavior. *Nursing Research, 48,* 29-34.

Youngblut, J. M., Loveland-Cherry, C. J., & Horan, M. (1991). Maternal employment effects on family and preterm infants at three months. *Nursing Research, 40,* 272-275.

Youngblut, J. M., Loveland-Cherry, C. J., & Horan, M. (1993). Maternal employment, family functioning, and preterm infant development at 9 and 12 months. *Research in Nursing & Health, 16,* 33-43.

Youngblut, J. M., Loveland-Cherry, C. J., & Horan, M. (1994). Maternal employment effects on families and preterm infants at 18 months. *Nursing Research, 43,* 331-337.

Youngblut, J. M., Singer, L. T., Madigan, E. A., Swegart, L. A., & Rodgers, W. L. (1997). Mother, child, and family factors related to employment of single mothers with LBW preschoolers. *Psychology of Women Quarterly, 21,* 247-263.

Youngblut, J. M., Singer, L. T., Madigan, E. A., Swegart, L. A., & Rodgers, W. L. (1998). Maternal employment and parent-child relationships in single-parent families of low birthweight preschoolers. *Nursing Research, 47,* 114-121.

EXEMPLAR STUDY 2:
IDENTIFICATION OF THE THEORETICAL FRAMEWORK

Sherman, D. W. (1996). Nurses' willingness to care for AIDS patients and spirituality, social support, and death anxiety. *Image, 28*(3), 205–213.

A. *The Science of Unitary Human Beings (SUHB) is used as the conceptual model.* The author supports the conceptualization of variables within the model by citing other theorists. For example,

Spirituality

— openness, personal integrity, wholeness (Helminiak)
— greater sense of awareness (Watson), transcendence (Ellison)

Transition into a life ever new

Death

AIDS

(human–environment diversity)

Courage   **Risk taking**   **Compassion**

Assumption :

— people find meaning in life and death, enhancing capacity to participate in change by exercising choices to fulfill potential

Conceptualizations:

— experience and awareness of human–environment integrity is conceptualized as spirituality, and perceived support (also are subscales)

B. *Literature (mainly theoretical) is cited as consistent with the SUHB.*

Creates need for care by others

Resistance

— **negative attitudes**	**WILLINGNESS TO CARE**	**Values**
— **RNs**		— **humanitarian obligation to others**
— **faculty**		
— **students**		
Spirituality	**Moral decision**	**Perceived support**
	— **mortality**	
	— **fear of death**	

93

Nurses' Willingness to Care for AIDS Patients and Spirituality, Social Support, and Death Anxiety

Deborah Witt Sherman

Objective: Use Rogers' (1992) framework of the science of unitary human beings to examine relationships among spirituality, perceived social support, death anxiety, and nurses' willingness to care for AIDS patients.

Design: Descriptive, correlational.

Population, Sample, Setting: Population, female RNs in the New York City Metropolitan area who care for patients with AIDS. Convenience sample of 220 RNs who worked in eight hospitals either on AIDS-dedicated units (n = 88), or medical-surgical scatterbed units (n = 132) with a daily AIDS patient census of between 5% to 50%. Data were collected in 1992.

Measures: Spiritual Orientation Inventory, the Personal Resource Questionnaire-85, the Templer Death Anxiety Scale, and the Willingness to Care for AIDS Patients Instrument.

Methods: Pearson product-moment correlations and hierarchical multiple regression analyses to test hypotheses.

Findings: Willingness to care for AIDS patients was positively correlated with spirituality and perceived social support, and negatively correlated with death anxiety. Death anxiety moderated the relationship between spirituality and willingness to care. In total, 17% of the variance in nurses' willingness to care for AIDS patients was explained. Additional regression analyses indicated that group membership as either an AIDS-dedicated nurse or medical-surgical nurse did not moderate or change hypothesized relationships.

Conclusion: Because group membership explained 22% of the variance in willingness to care, the data indicate that group culture or professional identity should be further examined as predictors of nurses' willingness to care for AIDS patients.

Clinical Implications: Social support at work from administrators and colleagues, as well as the support from patients themselves is important to nurses and should be fostered.

IMAGE: JOURNAL OF NURSING SCHOLARSHIP, 1996; 28(3), 205-213. ©1996, SIGMA THETA TAU INTERNATIONAL.

[Keywords: AIDS; willingness to care; spirituality; perceived social support; death anxiety]

*   *   *

Acquired immunodeficiency syndrome (AIDS) is a transmissible and universally fatal disease of epidemic proportions (Cohen, Sande, & Volberding, 1990). Several studies have indicated the resistance of some professional nurses and nursing students to providing AIDS care (Ficarrotto et al., 1989; Morgan & Treadway, 1989), despite AIDS education (Williams, Benedict, & Pearson, 1992). The negative attitudes of professionals are of concern for many reasons. First, AIDS patients are vulnerable (Hutton, 1987), and negative attitudes may result in patients' needless suffering (Morgan & Treadway, 1989). Second, the nurses' refusal to care for patients with AIDS shunts the responsibility to others, thereby increasing their risk of exposure (Huerta & Oddi, 1992).

According to Loewy (1988), the willingness to care for AIDS patients involves moral choices. Confronted with their own mortality (Bolle, 1988; Scanlon & Packard, 1991) and vulnerability (Flauskerud, 1987; Meisenhelder & LaCharite, 1989), nurses may experience the fear of death or death anxiety in providing AIDS care. Because spirituality is a way of being or experiencing characterized by a coherent system of life values

(Elkins, Hedstrom, Hughes, Leaf, & Saunders, 1988), and because perceived social support provides a sense of alliance in stressful situations (Weiss, 1974), both spirituality and perceived social support may also be corollaries to nurses' willingness to care for AIDS patients. The purpose of this descriptive, correlational study was to investigate the relationships among death anxiety, spirituality, perceived social support, and nurses' willingness to care for patients with AIDS.

Theoretical Framework

Rogers' science of unitary human beings (1970, 1986, 1987, 1990, 1992) provided the framework. Within the Rogerian framework, the AIDS epidemic may be viewed as an example of human-environmental diversity that demands courage, risk-

Deborah Witt Sherman, RN, PhD, *Upsilon*, is Assistant Professor of Nursing, Division of Nursing, School of Education, New York University, New York. Correspondence to Dr. Sherman, R.D. #3 Box 422, Fort Hill Road, Goshen, NY 10924.

Accepted for publication May 16, 1995

Note. From "Nurses Willingness to Care for AIDS Patients and Spirituality, Social Support, and Death Anxiety," by D. W. Sherman, 1996, *Image*, 28 pp. 205–213. Copyright 1996 by Blackwell Publishing, LTD. Reprinted with permission.

taking, and compassion (Rogers, 1992). The science of unitary human beings offers a paradigm from which one can derive theories that describe a phenomenon of concern, such as nurses' willingness to care for AIDS patients. In this study, it was theorized that a person's experience and awareness of integrality with the environment promotes a conceptualization of self beyond a physical dimension, infinite with the universe, and supports the view of death not as an end state but as a transition into life ever new (Reeder, 1990). People thus find meaning in life and death, enhancing their capacity to participate in change by exercising choices in fulfillment of their potential (Rogers, 1970). The experience and awareness of human-environmental integrality was conceptualized as spirituality and perceived social support. The interpretation of death was conceptualized as death anxiety. It was hypothesized that spirituality, perceived social support, and death anxiety would be related to a nurse's choice in fulfilling nursing potential, made evident by a willingness to care for AIDS patients.

Literature Review

Willingness to Care for AIDS Patients

Understanding the willingness or unwillingness of nurses to care for patients with AIDS involves the concept of will. For centuries, the idea of will has been debated from philosophical, theological, and psychoanalytical perspectives. Although Rogers (1970) did not discuss the will or willingness, she wrote that people possess a capacity to perceive relationships that is basic to organized action, and is identifiable by knowing participation in the patterning of the human-environmental field. Congruent with Rogers' views (1990), Assagioli (1973) believes that it is our dynamic, inner energy that makes us "willing," and that through awareness of self and the world, a person perceives power to choose, relate, and bring about changes in self, others, and circumstances. Because the will is guided by spiritual values, the act of being willing is consistent with the welfare of others and the good of humanity.

Barrick (1986) defined willingness to care for patients with AIDS as a relative readiness and absence of reluctance to care for them, and operationalized this definition in the Willingness to Care for AIDS Patients' Instrument, used in this study. The unwillingness or reluctance of many nurses to care for people with AIDS has been reported in several studies (Bond et al., 1990; Kelly, St. Lawrence, Smith, Hook, & Cook, 1988; Kerr & Horrocks, 1990). In a study of health care workers, Gordin and colleagues (1987) found that nurses ($n = 505$) were least willing to volunteer to work on AIDS units and one-third believed they should be able to refuse to care for patients with AIDS. Wiley, Earl, and Barnard (1990) found that over half the nurses ($n = 323$) studied would refuse an AIDS-related assignment if given the option and nearly one-third considered changing their profession because of the AIDS risk. In a 4-year longitudinal study, Scherer, Haughey, Wu, and Miller (1992) examined the attitudes of 552 and 567 RNs, respectively, from Erie County, New York, and found that negative attitudes toward AIDS patients persisted.

Such responses have also been found in studies of nursing students. Lester and Beard (1988) reported that in a sample of 177 baccalaureate nursing students, only one-third were willing to care for patients with AIDS. Wiley, Heath, and Acklin (1988) indicated that 21% of masters' nursing students ($n = 47$), 40% of RN/BSN students (n = 18), and 45% of undergraduate students ($n = 77$) would definitely or probably refuse to care for patients with AIDS. Based on a sample ($n = 166$) of four levels of nursing students and faculty, Oermann and Gignac (1991) found that faculty scores on attitude and willingness to care for AIDS patients were similar to those of students even though faculty scored highest on knowledge about AIDS. The authors concluded that willingness to care for patients with AIDS requires not only a base of knowledge needed to care but also attitudes and values that create greater willingness.

Spirituality

Consistent with the Rogerian perspective, spirituality is characterized by Helminiak (1987) as the openness, personal integrity, and wholeness of a person, which is tied to a greater sense of awareness (Watson, 1988), and to transcendence (Ellison, 1983). According to Brightman (1942), spirituality is a conscious experience involving knowing, willing, and growing in scope and power.

Malinski (1991) defined spirituality as the existence and experience of human-environmental integrality, of interconnection that involves pandimensional forms of awareness and facilitates knowing participation in change, and the ability of human beings to transcend reality. Consistent with Rogers' (1992) world view, Elkins, Hedstrom, Hughes, Leaf, and Saunders (1988) defined spirituality as "A way of being and experiencing that comes about through the awareness of a transcendent dimension and is characterized by certain identifiable values in regard to self, others, nature, life, and whatever one considers to be Ultimate" (p. 10). Spirituality optimizes the human potential: It involves awareness of a transcendent dimension, meaning and purpose in life, mission, altruism, idealism, awareness of the tragic, and a belief in the sacredness of life (Elkins et al., 1988).

Scanlon and Packard (1991) believe that AIDS caregivers who are well rooted in a value system and feel a connectedness with others, enjoy greater personal satisfaction in their work and thus potentially manifest greater willingness to continue such work. In examining the motivation of AIDS volunteers, Synder and Omoto (1992) concluded that willingness to care for patients with AIDS was related to their personal values, described as humanitarian obligation to help others, and community concern.

Perceived Social Support

In Rogers' view (1990), manifestations of human-environmental patterns arise from human-environmental integrality. Barrett (1990) suggests that one such manifestation is interpersonal relationships. Perceived social support is recognized as a measure of interpersonal relationships that provide environmental resources integral to a person's health, well-being, and social functioning (Cohen & Syme, 1985; Wortman, 1984), especially in major life roles (Kahn &

Antonucci, 1980). Social support has also been described as a dynamic phenomenon of "patterns of perceiving and interacting with the environment" (Broadhead et al., 1983, p. 531), "as the cognitive appraisal of being reasonably connected with others" (Barrera, 1986, p. 416), and as a simultaneous person-environment fit in which needs and abilities of a person are matched with resources and demands of the environment (Kahn, 1979).

Weiss (1974), in his theory of social support, proposed that interpersonal relationships offer attachment in which an individual experiences a personal commitment, social integration involving the sharing of ideas, opportunity for nurturance and nurturant behavior, reassurance of worth, and a sense of reasonable alliance that overcomes a sense of vulnerability.

Within the context of AIDS care, the perception of social support may strengthen a person's morale in difficult situations (Gottlieb, 1983); support the adoption of appropriate roles and behaviors (Thoits, 1982); and empower with information, self-esteem, and the resources necessary to exercise choices and to knowingly participate in change (Barrett, 1990). As such, the perception of social support is recognized as important in enhancing nurses' caregiving potential to patients with AIDS (Bolle, 1988; Scanlon & Packard, 1991). A lack of support from family and friends has been related to nurses' reluctance or refusal to provide AIDS care (Blumenfield, Smith, Milazzo, Seropian, & Wormser, 1987; O'Dowd, 1991).

Death Anxiety

According to Rogers (1970), people are aware of their mortality and seek a personal meaning of death. From a reductionistic perspective of the universe as primarily physical and material, death has been viewed as a degenerative physical and mental process (Hine, 1982). Even more threatening is death as punishment, with bodily mutilation and complete annihilation (Rheingold, 1967; Walton, 1979). These perceptions of death evoke death anxiety, defined "as an unpleasant emotional feeling upon contemplation of one's own death" (Lonetto & Templer, 1986).

In contrast, Rogers (1970, 1992) conceives of death as a dynamic patterning in which the human energy field moves "beyond the visible wave frequencies of the human field pattern that can be perceived by the human eye" (Phillips, 1990, p. 20). Taking Rogers' perspective, Schorr (1983) proposed that people who are aware of their integrality with the environment, and of self as a being, more than as a mere bodily structure, accept death without fear. Death is considered a part of life and is viewed as an alteration between two states of being, one constrained by the physical body and one free.

Nurses' personal perceptions related to death have been found to influence their attitudes, beliefs, and behaviors, and the types of interaction they have with terminally ill patients (Brockopp, King, & Hamilton, 1991; Hare & Pratt, 1989; Stoller, 1981). In explaining the unwillingness to care for patients with AIDS, death anxiety has been identified as a probable factor associated with health professionals' negative responses (Wyald & Cappel, 1990). Gordon (1970) and Mayer (1989) suggested that fear of death leads to reactive behavior. In relation to AIDS, fear of death

may engender behavior characterized by avoidance (Mayer, 1989; Momeyer, 1985), extreme precaution, and lack of regard for those affected (Flaskerud, 1989).

The hypotheses and research questions were derived from Rogers' conceptual framework and a review of the literature. The hypotheses were (a) There is a positive relationship between spirituality and nurses' willingness to care for patients with AIDS, independent of perceived social support and death anxiety; (b) There is a positive relationship between perceived social support and nurses' willingness to care for patients with AIDS, independent of spirituality and death anxiety; and (c) There is a negative relationship between death anxiety and nurses' willingness to care for patients with AIDS, independent of spirituality and perceived social support.

The research questions were as follows. Does death anxiety moderate the relationship between spirituality and nurses' willingness to care for patients with AIDS? Does death anxiety moderate the relationship between perceived social support and nurses' willingness to care for patients with AIDS? Are the hypothesized relationships different based on group membership?

Methods

Participants

The population of interest was female RNs from eight medical centers in the New York City metropolitan area who provided care for patients with AIDS. Participants were accrued over an 8-week period in 1992 from both AIDS-dedicated units and medical-surgical units with a daily AIDS patient census ranging from 5% to 50%. Following a description of the study, the nurses of the AIDS units and respective medical-surgical units were invited to participate. If they agreed, they were given the questionnaire packet, which they returned by mail. The volunteer, convenience sample of 220 female RNs included 88 who had chosen to work on AIDS-dedicated units and 132 medical-surgical nurses. Calculating 30 subjects per predictor variable, the sample size of 220 was adequate to test not only the hypotheses and research questions but was appropriate to conduct additional analyses. The sample was limited to female RNs because the literature suggests that men differ from women concerning death anxiety and perceived social support (Kastenbaum, 1986; Norbeck, 1981).

Participants ranged from 21 to 69 years of age with 71% in their 20s or 30s. The highest percentage of nurses was White (40%), followed by Asian (29%), Black (19.5%), and Hispanic (5.5%). Most (98%) were heterosexual; 40% were married; 42% were never married; and more than half (58%) did not have children. Most (68%) reported being very religious or somewhat religious and expressed belief in an afterlife; 56% were Catholic; 20% were Protestant; 21% were of an Eastern philosophy; and 3% were Jewish. All rated their health as moderately good to excellent.

The number of years as an RN ranged from 1 to 42, with 57% reporting from 2 to 10 years of nursing experience. Half (51%) indicated that their highest level of education was a baccalaureate degree in nursing or other field, 24% reported an associate degree in nursing, 15% were diploma graduates, 5% were masters' prepared, and 5% reported "other" degrees. Nearly all (95%) were full-time employees, with 62% working either an 8- or 12-hour daytime shift, and 38% working the evening or night shift. Although 20% held supervisory positions, all the nurses provided direct patient care. Nearly 60% reported they provide care to an equivalent number of intravenous drug users and homosexuals; an overwhelming majority (90%) expressed average to above average satisfaction with their work.

Instruments

Participants completed a self-administered questionnaire in booklet form that included the following instruments: The Willingness to Care for AIDS Patients Instrument (WCAPI) (Barrick, 1986), the Spiritual Orientation Inventory (SOI) (Elkins, 1988), the Personal Resource Questionnaire-85 (PRQ-85) (Brandt & Weinert, 1981; Weinert, 1987), and the Templer Death Anxiety Scale (TDAS) (Templer, 1970). A demographic information sheet was also included.

The Willingness to Care for AIDS Patients Instrument (Barrick, 1986) consists of six randomly ordered "willingness" questions that are combined with buffer questions to produce a 13-item instrument with a nine-point Likert scale. Higher scores on the instrument indicate greater "unwillingness" to care. Based on two pilot studies and a research study conducted by Barrick (1986), Cronbach's alpha coefficients of .77, .86, and .71 were computed, respectively. The Cronbach's alpha coefficient in the current study was .77. Content validity was established by a panel of AIDS educators and clinicians. Criterion validity was established based on a group of clinical nurses who chose to work exclusively with patients who had AIDS. As expected, their scores were at the extreme low end of the scale indicating their high willingness to provide AIDS care (Barrick, 1986).

The Spiritual Orientation Inventory (Elkins et al., 1988) was developed based on humanistic perspectives of spirituality and interviews of highly spiritual members of five religious traditions. The nine subscales of the SOI include: Awareness of a transcendent dimension, meaning and purpose in life, mission in life, belief in the sacredness of life, material values, altruism, idealism, awareness of the tragic, and fruits of spirituality; 85 items are responded to on a seven-point Likert scale. Higher scores represented greater spirituality. Reliability was established based on a sample of 96 participants; alpha coefficients ranged from .75 to .95 for the subscales (Elkins et al., 1988). In this study, the total alpha coefficient for the scale was .97, indicating a high level of internal consistency. The alpha coefficients of the subscales ranged from .72 to .95, with the exception of the subscale, Awareness of the Tragic, which had a low coefficient of .55. Content validity was established by five experts in psychology and spirituality. Criterion validity was established by comparing the scores of 96 graduate students in psychology with 24 participants nominated by a panel as highly spiritual persons.

Perceived social support was measured by the Personal Resource Questionnaire-85 (Brandt & Weinert, 1987). As a two-part multidimensional instrument, it is based on Weiss' (1974) five dimensions of social relationships: Provisions of attachment, social integration, opportunity for nurturance, worth, and assistance. Part 1, which is a description of situational support,

was not used in this study. Part 2, which was used, consists of 25 items with a Likert seven-point response format. Weinert (1987) established the reliability of the PRQ-85 based on three different samples of middle-aged to older adults; alpha coefficients ranged from .87 to .89. The alpha coefficient of the current study was .89. Construct validity of the PRQ-85 was established by a correlation of .58 with the Cost and Reciprocity Index, a new index of social support. Assessments of criterion validity have included moderate negative correlations with the Profile of Mood States ($r = -.31$, $p < .05$) and Beck Depression Inventory ($r = -.48$, $p < .05$).

The Templer Death Anxiety Scale (Templer, 1970), one of the most widely used measures of conscious death anxiety (Martin, 1982), consists of 15 true or false items, with scores ranging from 0 to 15. Higher scores indicate higher death anxiety. Based on a sample of 31 college students, test-retest reliability after 3 weeks was .83. A coefficient of .76 (Kuder-Richardson Formula 20) demonstrated reasonable internal consistency with these 31 students' responses (Templer, 1970). As reports on the reliability of the TDAS based on nursing samples were not evident in the literature, a pilot study was conducted using a sample of 30 nurses enrolled in a doctoral course. A reliability coefficient of .78 was computed. In the current study, the TDAS's reliability was computed at .63, certainly lower than was anticipated based on the results of the pilot study. Criterion validity was demonstrated by Templer (1970) on a group of psychiatric patients who were regarded as highly anxious. Construct validity was evident by significant correlations with Boyar's Fear of Death Scale, $r = .74$, $p < .05$, and the Death Anxiety Questionnaire, $r = .51$, $p < .01$ (Conte, Weiner, & Plutchik, 1982).

Procedures

Following the study's approval by the institution's review board, nurse managers were consulted to identify an appropriate time to provide the staff with a verbal and written description of the study, including its purpose, the voluntary nature of participation, opportunity to withdraw from the study at any time, and agreement to the one-time completion of a questionnaire booklet requiring approximately 60 to 90 minutes. Anonymity was assured. Tacit consent was indicated by the mailed return of a completed questionnaire booklet. The survey design, which was based on the Dillman Total Design Method (Dillman, 1978), motivates participants to respond and facilitates questionnaire completion. The questionnaire return rate was 82%. Using SPSS/PC, all data were entered twice for verification. Statistical analyses were conducted using the Statistical Package for the Social Sciences (SPSS/PC+, Version 4.0), with the level of statistical significance set at .05.

Results

The means, standard deviations, possible and actual score ranges, and skew of the instruments are in **Table 1.** The scale mean of the WCAPI indicated that these RNs were moderately willing to care for patients with AIDS. Templer, Ruff, and Franks (1971) reported a mean on the death anxiety instrument ranging

Table 1: Means, Standard Deviations, Possible and Actual Score Ranges, and Skew of the Psychometric Instruments (N = 220)

Instrument	Scale Mean	Standard Deviation	Possible Range	Actual Range	Skew
Willingness to Care for AIDS Patients Instrument	20.9	10.6	6 - 54	6 - 54	.59
Templer Death Anxiety Scale	8.2	2.6	0 - 15	1 - 15	.08
Personal Resource Questionnaire-85	146.9	16.3	25 - 175	82 - 175	-.87
Spiritual Orientation Inventory	450.5	68.5	85 - 595	254 - 580	.25

from 4.5 to 7 with a standard deviation of about 3. The mean for this study's sample revealed a higher death anxiety than the average adult population and a slightly lower standard deviation. In evaluating the RN scores on the PRQ-85, the mean and standard deviation falls within the range reported by Weinert (1989). The mean on the SOI revealed that the RNs had a moderately high level of spirituality. As the skew of all instruments was less than one, transformation of the variables was not indicated before conducting parametric statistical procedures.

The first hypothesis predicted a positive relationship between spirituality and nurses' willingness to care for patients with AIDS, independent of perceived social support and death anxiety. Before conducting multivariate statistical analyses, such as hierarchical multiple regressions, zero-order correlations offered preliminary evidence of the magnitude and direction of the relationships between the predictors and criterion variable. A Pearson product-moment correlation indicated a statistically significant correlation between spirituality and nurses' willingness to care for patients with AIDS ($r = -.24$, $p < .001$). Because higher scores on the WCAPI indicates greater *unwillingness* to care, the negative coefficient is interpreted as the greater the nurses' spirituality, the greater the *willingness* to care, thereby supporting the predicted direction of the relationship. Since willingness to care for patients with AIDS was conceptualized within the Rogerian framework as a unitary phenomenon, it was important to statistically control for any shared variance among the predictors. A hierarchical regression analysis was thereby conducted to examine spirituality's unique contribution in explaining the variance in nurses' willingness to care for patients with AIDS (**Table 2**). To remove any shared variance spirituality

may have with the other predictors, perceived social support and death anxiety were entered together in the first step of the regression equation. When spirituality was entered in step two of the equation, the R^2 change (.024) was statistically significant (F [1, 216] = 6.1, $p = .01$), indicating that spirituality uniquely explained 2% of the variance in willingness to care for patients with AIDS. Hypothesis 1 was therefore supported.

The second hypothesis predicted a positive relationship between perceived social support and nurses' willingness to care for patients with AIDS, independent of spirituality and death anxiety. A Pearson product-moment correlation indicated a statistically significant relationship ($r = .25$, $p < .001$) between perceived social support and willingness to care. Again, this negative relationship can be attributed to the fact that higher scores on the WCAPI indicate greater *unwillingness* to care. The correlation is therefore interpreted as the greater the nurses' perceived social support, the greater the willingness to care. To examine the unique contribution of perceived social support in explaining willingness to care, a hierarchical regression analysis was conducted (**Table 3**). Spirituality and death anxiety were entered on step one of the equation to remove any shared variance with perceived social support. Perceived social support was then entered on step two of the equation. The R^2 change (.046) was statistically significant (F [1, 216] = 11.68, $p < .001$) and indicated that perceived social support uniquely contributed 5% to the variance in willingness to care. Hypothesis 2 was therefore supported.

The third hypothesis predicted a negative relationship between death anxiety and nurses' willingness to care for patients with AIDS, independent of spirituality and perceived social support. A Pearson product-moment correlation indicated a statistically significant relationship ($r = .23$, $p < .001$) between death anxiety and willingness to care. Based on the scoring of the WCAPI, the correlation supported the predicted relationship that the greater the nurses' death anxiety, the less the willingness to care for AIDS patients. A hierarchical regression analysis (Table 4) was performed to examine the unique contribution of death anxiety in explaining willingness to care. Spirituality and perceived social support were entered in step one. Death anxiety was then entered in step two of the equation. The R^2 change (.04) was statistically significant (F [1,216] = 10.44, $p < .001$) and indicated that death anxiety accounted for 4% of the variance in willingness to care. Hypothesis 3 was supported.

A research question asked if low or high death anxiety changes the strength or direction of the relationship between spirituality and

Table 2: Hierarchical Multiple Regression Examining the Unique Contribution of Spirituality in Explaining Nurses' Willingness to Care for AIDS Patients (N = 220)

Step	Variable Entered	Multiple R	R^2	R^2 Change	Beta	F Change df = 3,216	Signif. F Change
1	Death Anxiety						
	Perceived Social Support	.345	.119	.119		14.68	< .001
2	Spirituality	.378	.143	.024	-.16	6.10	.014

Table 3: Hierarchical Multiple Regression Examining the Unique Contribution of Perceived Social Support in Explaining Nurses' Willingness to Care for AIDS Patients (N = 220)

Step	Variable Entered	Multiple R	R^2	R^2 Change	Beta	F Change df = 3,216	Signif. F Change
1	Death Anxiety Spirituality	.311	.097	.097		11.66	< .001
2	Perceived Social Support	.378	.143	.046	-.22	11.68	< .001

Step	Variable Entered	Multiple R	R^2	R^2 Change	Beta	F Change df = 3,216	Signif. F Change
1	Spirituality						
	Perceived Social Support	.319	.10	.10		12.32	< .001
2	Death Anxiety	.378	.143	.04	.21	10.44	< .001

Table 4: Hierarchical Multiple Regression Examining the Unique Contribution of Death Anxiety in Explaining Nurses' Willingness to Care for AIDS Patients (N = 220)

nurses' willingness to care for patients with AIDS. Spirituality and death anxiety were entered together in step one of a hierarchical regression analysis. The moderating variable was computed by multiplying spirituality by death anxiety and it was entered on step two of the regression equation. The R^2 change of the moderating variable was statistically significant (F [1, 216] = 8.06, p = .005) and accounted for 3% of the variance in nurses' willingness to care. Because the contribution of the moderating variable was statistically significant, a median split was then performed to divide death anxiety scores into low and high. In the presence of low death anxiety, a Pearson product-moment correlation indicated a nearly moderate, statistically significant relationship (r = -.29, p < .001) between spirituality and nurses' willingness to care. Remember that the negative sign of the coefficient resulted from the scoring of the WCAPI because higher scores indicate greater "unwillingness" to care. Thus, the negative direction of the relationship was interpreted as the higher the nurses' spirituality, the greater the willingness to care for AIDS patients. In the presence of high death anxiety, the correlation coefficient revealed a weaker relationship between the variables (r = -.14, p < .001). This indicated that death anxiety moderated the relationship between spirituality and nurses' willingness to care.

A second research question was whether death anxiety moderated the relationship between perceived social support and nurses' willingness to care for AIDS patients. The results of a hierarchical regression analysis determined that the moderating variable (death anxiety X perceived social support) was not statistically significant (F [1, 216] = .88, p = .34). Because death anxiety did not moderate or change the magnitude or direction of the relationship between the perceived social support and nurses' willingness to care for patients with AIDS, no further computations were necessary.

In total, 17% of the variance in willingness to care for AIDS patients was explained by the three predictors in the regression equation: spirituality, perceived social support, and death anxiety, along with the moderating variable of death anxiety times spirituality.

In addition, the third research question examined differences in the hypothesized relationships based on group membership as either AIDS-dedicated nurses or medical-surgical nurses. To conduct such analyses, a group membership variable was computed with AIDS-dedicated nurses dummy coded as group 0 and the medical-surgical nurses as group 1. The effect of group membership as a moderating variable was examined in relation to each of the three hypotheses with willingness to care as the

criterion variable. In three separate regression analyses, the group membership variable and the specific predictor, as either spirituality, perceived social support, or death anxiety, were entered together on step one of the regression equation. The moderating variable was then computed by multiplying the group membership variable by the specific predictor, which was then entered on step two of each equation. The results of the regression analyses indicated that R^2 change of each of the respective moderating variables was .00, and the associated p values were greater than the accepted .05 level of statistical significance, and therefore were not statistically significant. It was thus evident that group membership as either an AIDS-dedicated or medical-surgical nurse did not change the hypothesized relationships. It was interesting to note, however, that the group membership variable did explain 22% of the variance in nurses' willingness to care for AIDS patients.

Discussion

Statistical support of the three hypotheses provided preliminary validity for the propositions derived from both the science of unitary human beings and the literature review. The writings of Arendt (1978), Kane (1981), and May (1982) supported the relationship of the spirit and will either with the will as the instrument of the spirit or as designating movements of the spirit. Vaughan's (1991) conceptualization of spirituality as authenticity of thoughts, feelings, and actions; facing our fears to reduce anxiety; love and compassion; sense of community indicated by altruistic values; and liberation from excessive self-concern strongly suggested a relationship between spirituality and nurses' willingness to care for AIDS patients. Bolle (1988) and Scanlon and Packard (1991) also proposed that the spiritual values of nurses may be important in the care of patients with AIDS. Consistent with predictions in the literature, the relationship between spirituality and nurses' willingness to care was statistically supported, yet the modest correlations of the variables leads to further reflection. Nurses' willingness to care for patients with AIDS may be related not only to nurses' personal values and beliefs, as expressed by spirituality, but also to their professional identity and the associated role expectations. Siminoff, Erlen, and Lidz (1991) suggested that nurses' professional socialization may clarify role expectations and norms and diffuse nurses' fears of patients with AIDS, thereby decreasing their reluctance to provide care. Indeed, Arnold (1989) proposed that as nurses sharpen their awareness of self, their spiritual frames of reference develop and the meaning of professional practice and actions are considered. It is therefore recommended that the relationship between spiritual values and professional identity and socialization be examined, as well as their roles as possible covariates in nurses' willingness to care.

In the literature, the value of social support was postulated as a factor in promoting the adoption of appropriate roles and behaviors (Thoits, 1982), in strengthening of morale in difficult situations (Gottlieb, 1983), and in promoting nurses' caregiving potential in the care of patients with AIDS (Bolle, 1988; Pasacreta & Jacobsen, 1989). The result of this study offers empirical support for the relationship between perceived social support and nurses' willingness to care for AIDS patients, yet greater variance in willingness to care might have been explained if the instrument were more specific rather than global, as operationalized by the PRQ-85. For example, conversations with study participants revealed that perceived work support provided by colleagues and hospital administrators was an important factor in promoting their willingness to care.

One AIDS-dedicated nurse wrote, "As nurses, we support each other so that we can focus on our professional rather than personal behavior...." In discussing why nurses actively seek a position on the AIDS-dedicated unit at John Hopkins University Hospital, the staff emphasized the importance of a family-like atmosphere in which staff members care for each other, as well as the value of administrative support, which enhances enthusiasm and makes work with AIDS patients a positive experience (American Health Consultants, 1992).

In addition, a focus on the value of professional support groups may further explain nurses' willingness to care because support groups are recognized for improving communication, decreasing isolation, decreasing anxiety, improving self-esteem, and enhancing morale (Pasacreta & Jacobsen, 1989). An instrument such as the Perceived Social Support for Caregiving Scale (Goodman, 1991) which measures, for example, the understanding, information, advice, and insight offered by support groups, may provide a better gauge of nurses' perceived social support in the hospital setting. One other source of social support that should also be considered is the possible support offered by patients themselves. From a Rogerian perspective, Boguslawski (1990) wrote that the mutual process between one individual and another is a powerful presence and energy that supports confidence, patience, and perseverance. This may explain the empirical evidence that the greater the contact with patients with AIDS, the greater the nurses' comfort and willingness to care for them (Jemmott, Jemmott III, & Cruz-Collins, 1992; Klisch, 1990; Synoground & Kellmer-Langan, 1991).

This study's finding concerning the negative relationship between death anxiety and nurses' willingness to care for patients with AIDS supports the theoretical proposition that the fear of death paralyzes action (Lepp, 1968) and limits one's ability to make responsible choices and to relate lovingly and freely with others (Maddi, 1980). This finding is also consistent with previous empirical studies that reported negative relationships between death anxiety and empathy for others (Westman & Canter, 1985) and tolerance for others (Vargo & Black, 1984). Though lower in magnitude, this study's finding is consistent with the negative relationship between fear of death and antipathy to the care of AIDS patients ($r = -.45$, $p < .05$) expressed by a sample of senior medical students (Merrill, Luax, & Thornby, 1989) and is consistent with the direction and magnitude of correlations reported between death anxiety and nurses' attitudes or behaviors in caring for the terminally ill (Hare & Pratt, 1989; Stoller, 1981; Thompson, 1986).

With regard to research question one, it was found that direct associations not only existed between the variables but that an interaction or moderating effect existed between death anxiety and spirituality that accounted for 3% of the variance in

willingness to care and changed the magnitude of the relationship between spirituality and nurses' willingness to care. High death anxiety weakened the correlation between spirituality and nurses' willingness to care.

Zukav (1989) explains that fear limits our perception to a five-sensory modality and that an individual with limited awareness has diminished strength of soul. Zukav's theory offers insight into the possible moderating effect of death anxiety. It may be that individuals with high death anxiety are limited in their experience and awareness of integrality with the environment. With the spirit weakened by fear, nurses cannot participate in liberating families and groups from the negativities of AIDS, hence their lessened willingness to care. Indeed, a profile of low death anxiety, heightened spirituality, and greater willingness to care may be a profile of nurses who knowingly participate in change by actualizing their nursing potential and accept their social responsibility or caring for patients with AIDS.

For the second research question, results indicated that there was no statistically significant relationship between death anxiety and perceived social support ($r = -.001$, $p = .49$), nor an interaction effect between the variables. Death anxiety therefore did not moderate the relationship between perceived social support and nurses' willingness to care for AIDS patients.

For the third research question, there were no differences in the hypothesized relationships based on group membership as either AIDS-dedicated or medical-surgical nurses. These findings provided an internal replication of the study and supported the hypothesized relationships among the variables. Because this study's sample included nurses who provided care in areas with a relatively high incidence of patients with AIDS, a focus of future research might be to compare the hypothesized relationships between nurses who work in areas with a high incidence of AIDS and those who work in areas with a low incidence. Given also that group membership as an AIDS-dedicated nurse explained 22% of the variance in nurses' willingness to care for AIDS patients, concepts such as group culture or professional identity should be examined in future studies as possible correlates to willingness to care.

Although the findings supported the theory derived from Rogers' Science of Unitary Human Beings and relationships among the variables postulated in the literature, the modest strength of the relationships leaves one to question whether the findings truly represent reality or can be attributed to conceptual issues or measurement error. For example, Barrick's (1986) definition of willingness to care, as a relative readiness or absence of reluctance to care for patients with AIDS, provided a narrow conceptualization. Because the theoretical literature addresses social responsibility, humanitarian action, the choice to do good, and risk-taking as dimensions of willing, the development of an instrument that incorporates such dimensions in measuring willingness to care for patients with AIDS may more completely capture the phenomenon of willingness and result in stronger correlations among the variables.

Although the Templer Death Anxiety Scale is often cited in the literature, the low reliability of the scale supports the recommendation that the instrument be pilot-tested on the specific sample to which it will be administered. The low reliability of the TDAS may be related to the forced true-or-false response format, which limited the response possibilities for each question. It is therefore suggested that a Likert response format, which offers a broader range of responses, may allow a researcher to better detect the real feelings of an individual.

One must also question whether stronger relationships would have been found if the sample of nurses was more heterogenous in its experience of caring for patients with AIDS. Although the intent of this research was to examine corollaries of willingness to care among nurses who were actively caring for patients with AIDS, the narrow range of their responses may have also contributed to the weaker correlations. These conceptual and methodological issues are important in replicating this study.

References

American Health Consultants (1992). U.S. residents have negative attitudes toward AIDS patients. **AIDS Alert, 7(10)**, 152-154.

Arendt, H. (1978). **The life of the mind: Two/Willing**. New York: Harcourt Brace Jovanovich.

Arnold, E. (1989). Burnout as a spiritual issue: Rediscovering meaning in nursing practice. In V. Carson (Ed.), **Spiritual dimensions of nursing practice** (320-353). Philadelphia: Saunders.

Assagioli, R. (1973). The act of will. New York: Penguin Books. Barrera, M. (1986). Distinction between social support concepts, measures, and models. **American Journal of Community Psychology, 14**, 413-445.

Barrett, E.A.M. (1990). **Visions of Rogers' science-based nursing**. New York: National League of Nursing.

Barrick, W. (1986). A correlational study of attitudes toward homosexuals and willingness to care for acquired immunodeficiency patients among nursing personnel. Master's thesis. San Francisco State University, California.

Blumenfield, M., Smith, P.J., Milazzo, J., Seropian, S., & Wormser, G.P. (1987). Survey of attitudes of nurses working with AIDS patients. **General Hospital Psychiatry, 9**, 58-63.

Bolle, J.L. (1988). Supporting the deliverers of care: Strategies to support nurses and prevent burnout. **Nursing Clinics of North America, 23**, 843-850.

Bond, S., Rhodes, T., Philips, P., Setters, J., Foy, C., & Bond, J. (1990). HIV infection and AIDS in England: The experience, knowledge and intentions of community nursing staff. **Journal of Advanced Nursing, 15**, 249-255.

Boguslawski, M. (1990). Unitary human field practice modalities. In E.A.M. Barrett (Ed.), **Visions of Rogers' science-based nursing** (93-104). New York: National League for Nursing.

Brandt, P.A., & Weinert, C. (1987). The PRQ: A social support measure. **Nursing Research, 30**, 277-280.

Brightman, E.S. (1942). **The spiritual life**. New York: Abingdon Cokesbury Press.

Broadhead, W.E., Kaplan, B.H., James, S.A., Wayne, E.H., Schoenback, V.J., Grimson, R., Heyden, S., Tibblin, G., & Gehlback, S.K. (1983). The epidemiologic evidence for a relationship between social support and health. **American Journal of Epidemiology, 117**, 521-537.

Brockopp, D.Y., King D.B., & Hamilton, J.E. (1991). The dying patient: A comparative study of nurse caregiver characteristics. **Death Studies, 15**, 245-258.

Cohen, P.T., Sande, M.A., & Volberding, P.A. (1990). The AIDS knowledge base. Waltham, MA: The Medical Publishing Group.

Cohen, S., & Syme, S.L. (1985). Social support and health. New York: Academic Press.

Conte, H.R., Weiner M.B., & Plutchik, R. (1982). Measuring death anxiety: Conceptual, psychometric, and factor analytic aspects. **Journal of Personality and Social Psychology, 43**, 775-785.

Dillman, D.A. (1978). **Mail and telephone surveys**. New York: John Wiley & Sons.

Elkins, D. (1988). **Spiritual Orientation Inventory**. (Available from D.N. Elkins, Ph.D., Pepperdine University Center, 2151 Michelson Drive, Suite 165, Irvine, CA, 92715.)

D., Hedstrom, L.J., Hughes, L., Leaf, J.A., & Saunders, C. (1988). Toward a humanistic-phenomenological spirituality. **Journal of Humanistic Psychology, 28(4)**, 5-18.

Ellison, C.W. (1983). Spiritual well-being: Conceptualization and measurement. **Journal of Psychology and Theology, 11**, 330-340.

Ficarrotto, T.J., Grade, M., Bartnof, H., Koenig, B., Bliwise, N., & Irish, T. (1989). Factors predictive of AIDS-HIV knowledge and attitudes among nursing and medical students. **International Conference on AIDS, 5**, 907.

Flaskerud, J.H. (1987). AIDS: Psychosocial aspects. **Journal of Psychosocial Nursing, 25(12)**, 9-16.

Flaskerud, J.H. (1989). **AIDS/HIV infection: A reference guide for nursing professionals**. Philadelphia: W.B. Saunders.

Goodman, C.C. (1991). Perceived social support for caregiving: Measuring the benefit of self-help/support group participation. **Journal of Gerontological Social Work, 16(3/4)**, 163-175.

Gordon, D. (1970). **Overcoming the fear of death**. New York: Macmillan.

Gottlieb, B.H. (1983). **Social support strategies**. Beverly Hills, CA: Sage Publications.

Hare, J., & Pratt, C. (1989). Nurses' fear of death and comfort level with dying patients. **Death Studies, 13**, 349-360.

Helminiak, D.A. (1987). Spiritual development. Chicago: Loyola University Press.

Hine, V. (1982). Holistic Dying: The role of the nurse clinician. **Topics in Clinical Nursing, 3**, 45-54.

Huerta, S.R., & Oddi, L.F. (1992). Refusal to care for patients with human immunodeficiency virus/acquired immunodeficiency syndrome: Issues and responses. **Journal of Professional Nursing, 8**, 221-230.

Hutton, M. (1987). AIDS and our attitudes-from a nursing perspective. **Journal of Palliative Care, 3(1)**, 48-49.

Jemmott, L.S., Jemmott III, J.B., & Cruz-Collins, M. (1992). Predicting AIDS patient care intentions among nursing students. **Nursing Research, 41**, 172-177.

Kahn, R.L. (1979). Aging and social support. In M.W. Riley (Ed.), Aging from birth to death-interdisciplinary perspective (77-91). Boulder, CO: Westview Press.

Kahn, R.L., & Antonucci, T. (1980). Convoys over the life course: Attachment, roles and social support. In P. Bates & O. Brim (Eds.), **Life span development and behavior** (253-288). New York: Academic Press.

Kane, G. (1981). **Anselm's doctrine of freedom and the will**. New York: Edwin Mallen Press.

Kastenbaum, R. (1986). Death, society and human experience. Columbus, OH: Charles E. Merrill Publishing.

Kelly, J.A., St. Lawrence, J.S., Smith, S., Hood, H., & Cook, D. J. (1988). Nurses attitudes toward AIDS. **Journal of Continuing Education in Nursing, 19(2)**, 78-83.

Kerr, C.I., & Horrocks, M.J. (1990). Knowledge, values, attitudes, and behavioral intent of Nova Scotia nurses toward AIDS and patients with AIDS. **Canadian Journal of Public Health, 81**, 125-128.

Klisch, M.L. (1990). Caring for persons with AIDS: Student reactions. **Nurse Educator, 15(4)**, 16-20.

Lepp, I. (1968). **Death and its mysteries**. New York: Macmillan.

Lester, L.B., & Beard, B.J. (1988). Nursing students attitudes towards AIDS. **Journal of Nursing Education, 27**, 399-404.

Loewy, E.H. (1988). Risk and obligation: Health professionals and the risk of AIDS. **Death Studies, 12**, 531-545.

Lonetto, R., & Templer, D.I. (1986). **Death anxiety**. Washington, DC: Hemisphere Publishing.

Maddi, S. (1980). Developmental value of fear of death. **The Journal of Mind and Behavior, 1(1)**, 85-92.

Malinski, V.M. (1991). Spirituality as integrality: A Rogerian perspective on the path of healing. **Journal of Holistic Nursing, 9(1)**, 54-64.

Martin, T. (1982). Death anxiety and social desirability among nurses. **Omega,** **13(1),** 51-58.

May, G. (1982). Will and spirit. New York: Harper Collins.

Mayer, D. (1989). Wholly life: A new perspective on death. **Holistic Nursing** **Practice, 3(4),** 72-80.

Meisenhelder, J.B., & LaCharite, C.L. (1989). Fear of contagion: A stress response to acquired immunodeficiency syndrome. **Advances in Nursing** **Science, 11(2),** 29-38.

Merrill, J., Laux, L., & Thornby, J. (1989). AIDS and student attitudes. **Southern Medical Journal, 82(4),** 426-432.

Momeyer, R. (1985). Fearing death and caring for the dying. **Omega, 16(1),** 1-9.

Morgan, K.J., & Treadway, J. (1989). Surveying nursing staff's attitudes about AIDS. **AIDS Patient Care, 9,** 35-39.

Norbeck, J.S. (1981). Social support: A model for clinical research and application. **Advances in Nursing Science, 3(4),** 43-59.

Norbeck, J.S. (1985). Types and sources of social support for managing job stress in critical care nursing. **Nursing Research, 34,** 225-230.

O'Dowd, M.A. (1991). Psychosocial issues and HIV. **AIDS Clinical Care, 3(11),** 81-83.

Oermann, M.H., & Gignac, D. (1991). Knowledge and attitudes about AIDS among Canadian nursing students: Educational implications. **Journal of** **Nursing Education, 30,** 217-221.

Pasacreta, J.V., & Jacobsen, P.B. (1989). Addressing the need for staff support among nurses caring for the AIDS population. **Oncology Nursing Forum,** **16,** 662-663.

Phillips, J.R. (1990). Changing human potentials and future visions of nursing: A human field image perspective. In E.A.M. Barrett (Ed.), **Visions of Rogers'** **science-based nursing,** (13-25)New York: National League of Nursing.

Reeder, F. (1990). Forward. In E.A.M. Barrett (Ed.), **Visions of Rogers' science-** **based nursing,** (xix). New York: National League of Nursing.

Rheingold, J. (1967). **The mother, anxiety, and death.** Boston: Little & Brown.

Rogers, M.E. (1970). **An introduction to the theoretical basis of nursing.** Philadelphia: F.A. Davis.

Rogers, M.E. (1986). Science of unitary human beings. In V.M. Malinski (Ed.), **Explorations on Martha Rogers' science of unitary human beings** (3-8). Norwalk, CT: Appleton-Century-Crofts.

Rogers, M.E. (1987). Rogers' science of unitary human beings. In R.R. Parse (Ed.), **Nursing science: Major paradigms, theories, and critiques** (139-146). Philadelphia: W.B. Saunders.

Rogers, M.E. (1990). Nursing: Science of unitary, irreducible, human beings: Update 1990. In E.A.M. Barrett (Ed.), **Visions of Rogers' science-based** **nursing** (5-11). New York: National League for Nursing.

Rogers, M.E. (1992). Nursing science and the space age. **Nursing Science** **Quarterly, 5(1),** 27-34.

Scanlon, C., & Packard, M. (1991). Seeing to one's self. **Health Progress,** **72(11),** 50-53.

Scherer, Y.K., Haughey, B.P., Wu, Y.W.B., & Miller, C.M. (1992). A longitudinal study of nurses' attitudes toward caring for patients with AIDS in Erie county. **Journal of the New York State Nurses Association, 23(3),** 10-15.

Schorr, J. (1983). Manifestations of consciousness and the developmental phenomenon of death. **Advances in Nursing Science, 6(1),** 27-35.

Siminoff, L., Erlen, J., & Lidz, C. (1991). Stigma, AIDS and quality of nursing care: State of the science. **Journal of Advanced Nursing, 16,** 262-269.

Stoller, E. (1981). The impact of death related fears on attitudes of nurses in a hospital work setting. **Omega, 11(1),** 85-96.

Synder, M., & Omoto, A.M. (1992). Volunteerism and society's response to the HIV epidemic. **Current Directions in Psychological Science, 1,** 113-116.

Synoground, S.G., & Kellmer-Langan, D.M. (1991). Nursing attitudes towards AIDS: Implications for education. **Nurse Education Today, 11,** 200-206.

Templer, D.I. (1970). The construction and validation of a death anxiety scale. **The Journal of General Psychology, 82,** 165-177.

Templer, D.I., Ruff, C., & Franks, C. (1971). Death anxiety: Age, sex, and parental resemblance in diverse populations. **Developmental Psychology, 4,** 108.

Thoits, P. (1982). Conceptual, methodological, and theoretical problems in studying social support as a buffer against life stress. **Journal of Health and** **Social Behavior, 10(23),** 145-159.

Thompson, E. (1986). Palliative and curative care nurses' attitudes toward dying and death in the hospital setting. **Omega, 16(3),** 233-241.

Vargo, M., & Black, F.W. (1984). Psychosocial correlates of death anxiety in a population of medical students. **Journal of Clinical Psychology, 40,** 1525-1528.

Vaughan, F. (1991). Spiritual issues in psychotherapy. **The Journal of** **Transpersonal Psychology, 23,** 105-119.

Walton, D. (1979). **On defining death.** London: McGill-Queen's University Press.

Watson, J. (1988). **Nursing: Human science and human care.** New York: National League for Nursing.

Weinert, C. (1987). A social support measure: PRQ85. **Nursing Research, 36,** 273-275.

Weinert, C. (1989). **Personal Resource Questionnaire-85: Summary of** **reliability estimates internal consistency.** Montana State University College of Nursing, Bozeman, MT.

Weiss, R.J. (1974). The provision of social relationships. In Z. Rubin (Ed.), **Doing unto others** (17-26). Eaglewood Cliffs, NJ: Prentice Hall.

Westman, A., & Canter, F. (1985). Fear of death and the concept of the extended self. **Psychological Reports, 56,** 419-425.

Wiley, K., Earl, A., & Barnard, B. (1990). Care of HIV-Infected patients: Nurses' concerns, opinions, and precautions. **Applied Nursing Research, 3(1),** 27-33.

Wiley, K., Heath, L., & Acklin, M. (1988). Care of AIDS patients: Student attitudes. **Nursing Outlook, 36,** 244-245.

Williams, R.D., Benedict, S., & Pearson, B.C. (1992). Degree of comfort in providing care to PWAs: Effect of a workshop for baccalaureate nursing students. **Journal of Nursing Education, 31,** 397-401.

Wortman, C.B. (1984). Social support and the cancer patient. **Cancer, 53,** 2339-2360.

Wyald, D., & Cappel, S. (1990). The big easy? Legal and managerial perspective on AIDS and health care delivery in the 1990s. **AIDS & Public Policy** **Journal, 5,** 99-106.

Zukav, G. (1989). **The seat of the soul.** New York: Simon & Shuster.

12

Guide to Critique of Qualitative Research with Examples and Practice Studies

These are questions to consider when critiquing a qualitative research study. Sample critiques and articles are included.

A. Title

1. Does the researcher indicate the focal topic and offer a metaphorical hint of interpretation?

B. Introduction

1. Is the phenomenon of interest explicitly identified and placed within a context?
2. Is the purpose of the inquiry clearly stated (e.g., discovery, theory building, descriptive base for practice, etc.?)
3. Is (are) the research question(s) broad and open ended or open beginning?
4. Has the researcher identified the significance of inquiring about this phenomenon, why it is important to study, and why it is important to use this method?
5. Is the researcher's context described (e.g., background, experiences, assumptions, preconceptions, beliefs about the phenomenon?)
6. What is the researcher's expertise in conducting this type of inquiry?

C. Literature Review and Theoretical Framework

1. If a literature review is appropriate to the method and prior to data collection, does it demonstrate the complexity of the phenomenon, provide additional justification and credence for the study. Does the summary of the literature signify how this inquiry will add to existing knowledge?

2.   If a theoretical perspective is used for the study, does it conform to the philosophic orientations and naturalistic axioms of qualitative research? Is the framework presented?

D.   Method

1.   Is there an overview of the qualitative method chosen, its philosophical underpinnings, and why it is appropriate for this study?
2.   Is there a thorough explication of the details—process and procedures—of the study?

E.   Sample—Participants

1.   Is the sampling procedure delineated? Is it appropriate for this inquiry?
2.   Are the participants, the setting, and the rationale for those chosen to be in the study described?
3.   Does the researcher discuss the process of gaining entrée to the setting (informal and official) and access to the participants?

F.   Data Collection

1.   Does the researcher identify the data collection techniques (e.g., interviews, participant observation, review of documents, etc.)? Are they appropriate for this study?
2.   Are the details and procedures of data collection explicated (e.g., how conducted, when, where, with whom, time per data collection sessions, saturation, tape recording, transcriber, training of data collectors, etc.)?
3.   Are informed consent and protection of human subjects in qualitative inquiry described?
4.   Are data records used during the study (transcripts, field notes, journals, logs) identified?
5.   Are problems in data collection, ethical issues, and researcher effects on the data discussed?

G.   Data Management and Analysis

1.   Does the researcher describe the plan for organizing and retrieving data?
2.   Does the researcher detail the processes and procedures for data analysis (e.g., coding, categorization, use of matrices, constant comparison, memoing, literature, software packages). Is a particular method of analysis identified? Is it appropriate for this study?
3.   If a framework were used, is it clear how it informed the analysis?
4.   Are the researcher's decision rules used to thematize the data made explicit?
5.   Are the researcher's interpretations, hypotheses, conclusions, or theoretical schema data based (e.g., supported or verified with substantive evidence and examples directly from the data)?

6. Is a clear, descriptive, contextual theoretical presentation of the meaning of the phenomenon as discovered by the researcher provided?
7. Is the work meaningful, giving voice to the participants and insights to the reader?

H. Discussion, Conclusions, Implications, Recommendations

1. Are the findings compared and contrasted with existing literature and theoretical perspectives?
2. Is there a comprehensive discussion of the results of the inquiry? Do the conclusions reflect the findings?
3. Does the researcher share his or her understanding and learning re: applications and/or implications as they influence present practices and understandings?
4. Are the relevance of the inquiry and the findings and the importance to nursing practice and knowledge building identified? Are they appropriate, based on the findings?
5. Are limitations of the study identified?
6. Are recommendations for further study and/or practice and/or education suggested?

I. Quality and Rigor of the Inquiry

1. Does the researcher address measures used to ensure trustworthiness of the inquiry (credibility, transferability, dependability, confirmability, ethics)?
2. Does the work possess verity, integrity, rigor, utility, vitality, and aesthetics? (see pp. 67–68)
3. Does the work have descriptive vividness, methodological congruence, analytic precision, theoretical connectedness, and heuristic relevance? (see pp. 67–68)
4. Does the work flow smoothly and offer the reader a sensitive, credible understanding of the human experience? Is it "real," "alive," and yet insightful?

EXEMPLAR STUDY 1 WITH CRITIQUE

Research article: Kosowski, M. M. and Roberts, V. W. (2003). When protocols are not enough: Intuitive decision making by novice nurse practitioners. *Journal of Holistic Nursing, 21*(1), 52–72.

A. Title

The focal topic of the study is indicated in the title (intuitive decision making by novice nurse practitioners) and a metaphorical hint of interpretation (insufficiency of protocols).

B. Introduction

The phenomenon of interest, novice nurse practitioners' intuitive decision making, is clearly identified and placed within a context of the national and rising demand for NPs in the twenty-first century, the need to educate NPs in a holistic framework, and the importance of intuition to complex decision making and the art and science of nursing. The purpose of the inquiry is clearly stated: "to discover, describe, and analyze the stories of novice NPs who use intuitive decision making with clients" (p. 112). The researchers identify the significance of the inquiry and the importance of using a qualitative approach by stating, "Whereas the literature addresses numerous barriers to practice form the perspective of scholars and researchers, NPs' perspectives on the problems they confront in everyday practice have not been examined in depth (Martin & Hutchinson, 1999). In addition, the literature is deficient in addressing the role of intuition . . . by NPs and resultant challenges to maintain holism and caring as the essence of their practices" (p. 111). The researchers' context is not discussed but can only be gleaned from the authors' credentials and academic orientation. There is no indication that the researchers have had prior expertise in conducting this type of inquiry.

C. Literature Review and Theoretical Framework

The literature review meets the criteria for demonstrating the complexity of the phenomenon, considering the page limit of most articles. Some of the references are dated and could be more recent. The literature review does provide justification for the study in both the last paragraph on p. 111 and throughout the **Methods Section** (p. 112). Two theoretical frameworks (feminist theory and postmodern perspectives), which are appropriate to the interpretative phenomenological method, were identified as guiding the inquiry. On p. 114 of the article the authors state that texts were "analyzed and examined from critical and feminist theory and postmodern perspectives to situate the stories within their political, social, and cultural contexts." This was not always clear in the presentation of the findings.

D. Methods

Kosowski and Roberts present a description of Interpretative Phenomenology, its purpose and major underlying assumption: "Interpretative phenomenology . . . bridges subjective and objective knowing by focusing on individual perceptions of phenomena and uncovering common themes and universals that emerge from narratives of persons' lived experiences (Tarzian, 2000) . . . this approach emphasizes the importance of everyday life experiences, multiple relativistic constructions of reality. . . . Therefore, to understand the experiences of NPs who used intuition in clinical decision making with clients, an interpretive phenomenological approach" was used (p. 112). The researchers explain the procedures of the study in the **Participants** section on pp. 112–113.

E. Sample—Participants

The researchers identified the participants in the study. Purposive sampling was used, which is appropriate for this type of study. The authors indicate who the participants were (10 recent graduates of a NP program), where the study was conducted, how the participants were informed of the study, and how the participants were chosen (purposive sampling until redundancy was reached). It would have been helpful if the total number of those willing to participate (several graduates) had been specifically identified and how those chosen to be in the study were selected. Brief demographics were included. Kosowski and Roberts do state that IRB approval was obtained from their institution.

F. Data Collection

The authors identified face-to-face confidential interviews as the data collection method. Pseudonyms were chosen by participants to enhance confidentiality. Some procedures and processes of data collection were used, including a reflexive dialectic feedback technique during the interviews to verify and clarify data collected, a tape recorder and transcription, interviews conducted at a time and place convenient for the participant, and follow-up with participants by mailing them a copy of their individual interviews to verify data accuracy and clarity. The prime question of the interview was identified by the authors. Length of the interviews, number of interviews per participant, and time between interviews were not discussed.

Kosowski and Roberts do not identify the types of data records, with the exception of interview transcripts used during the inquiry (e.g., interpretive notes, procedural notes and the purpose of each). Problems in data collection, potential ethical issues, and researcher effects (they are both from an academic institution and knew the participants as students for 5–10 years, p. 114) were not discussed.

G. Data Management and Analysis

The researchers identified use of the hermenutic analysis method of Diekelman and Allen (1989) to analyze the data. Kosowski and Roberts give a thorough description of the steps of this particular analytic method (e.g., reading of the texts for overall comprehension of meaning, summary, discussion for meaning and consensus, theme development linking meaning across texts, and identification of relationships among themes). Substantive evidence and examples from the interviews are given to support the analysis. As noted above, the frameworks (critical and feminist theory) from which the data were analyzed are not always apparent in the conceptualization of the interpretations.

Kosowski and Roberts present a constitutive process of NPs' use of intuition in clinical decision making containing six overlapping themes. These are: (1) reflecting, (2) backing it up, (3) knowing the rules, (4) playing the game, (5) learning lessons, and (6) taking care. The authors elucidate this process by describing in depth the various themes and the iterative nature of using intuition in clinical decision making. Each theme is discussed individually and verified, using excerpts from the participant interviews. The authors then provide a succinct narrative and a visual representation of the iterative constitutive pattern. The presentation of findings was clear, based in context, and supported by data-based examples.

H. Discussion, Conclusions, Implications, Recommendations

Kosowski and Roberts provide comparison of their findings with existing literature on RNs' need for reinforcement of intuition for holistic practice, literature supporting the need for NP education that includes critical thinking, intuitive decision making, and diverse patterns of knowing, and literature indicating that novice NPs be assisted through mentoring to maintain a holistic and caring philosophy to practice. The conclusions of the study reflect the findings as noted by comparison with the literature and that these NPs have a persistent struggle to maintain a holistic approach. Four recommendations for practice and education (i.e., nurturing and role modeling of intuition by faculty and preceptors, improved communications with physicians, support for NPs in maintaining a holistic orientation in practice, and need for all members of the profession to practice activities that enable holistic caring for self, clients, and colleagues) are provided by the investigators. The authors cite the relevance of the inquiry by emphasizing the increased numbers and responsibilities of NPs in health care and the significance of reflective, thoughtful, and intuitive decision making.

Kosowski and Roberts identify limitations of the study as a small, homogeneous sample; however, as the narratives were rich and deep, they have implications for NP practice. Four recommendations for further study are suggested: research with a larger sample, more diverse participants, triangulation of methods, and study of more experienced NPs.

L. Quality and Rigor of the Inquiry

On p. 114 of the **Data Analysis Section**, the researchers address measures to achieve trustworthiness of the study. These include credibility (member checking with participants for fairness and accuracy of interpretations, peer debriefing with a colleague who reviewed the summaries, themes and findings); confirmability (multiple member checks); transferability (purposive sampling and informational redundancy with rich, deep data and congruence of data across participants); and reporting a negative case.

Considering page limitations on most journals, the work as presented appears structurally sound, with a logical research rationale. The constitutive pattern of using intuition in clinical decision making is useful for understanding the experiences of novice NPs in maintaining holism and caring in their practice. It further gives us insights into the education of NPs and the challenges they face while transitioning into the NP role.

When Protocols Are Not Enough

Intuitive Decision Making by Novice Nurse Practitioners

Margaret M. Kosowski, R.N., Ph.D.
Vanice W. Roberts, R.N., D.S.N.
Kennesaw State University

The pressing need for health care reform in this century has contributed to an increasing interest in educating health care providers who can deliver cost-effective, high-quality care. Demand for primary care nurse practitioners has risen significantly, and nursing education has responded by increasing the numbers and graduates of nurse practitioner programs. Although this century brings new opportunities for expanded nursing roles, it also presents challenges for nurse practitioners to sustain a holistic perspective while providing quality care. The purpose of this interpretive phenomenological study was to discover, describe, and analyze the stories of 10 novice nurse practitioners who used intuition in clinical decision making. The authors maintained a critical social consciousness and postmodern perspective to analyze and describe the shared meanings and common practices of participants. This article discusses the six themes and constitutive process that emerged from the data and addresses implications for nurse practitioner education and practice.

Keywords: *nurse practitioners; intuition; clinical decision making; novice nurses; practice protocols*

In light of the pressing need for health care reform and the increasing numbers of uninsured and inadequately insured clients, there is widespread interest in educating health care providers who can deliver cost-effective, high-quality care for all Americans (Moser &

AUTHORS' NOTE: This research was partially funded by a scholar's grant from Sigma Theta Tau International Honor Society of Nursing Mu Phi Chapter.

JOURNAL OF HOLISTIC NURSING, Vol. 21 No. 1, March 2003 52-72
DOI: 10.1177/0898010102250275
© 2003 American Holistic Nurses' Association

Armer, 2000). Recently, the health care climate has embraced the primary care model, and nurse practitioners (NPs) with advanced education have been recognized as valuable members of health care teams (Adams & Miller, 2001). But the need for primary care NP providers is expected to rise significantly as managed care plans grow (Moore, 1994), and the demand for NPs will exceed its supply threefold early in the 21st century (Bezyack, 1996). Schools of nursing throughout the nation have responded to this need by revising curricula, reeducating faculty members, and increasing the number of primary care NP programs. The escalation of NP programs calls us to examine the adequacy of academic preparation for transitioning to the advanced practice role and for maintaining a holistic philosophy within these roles (Rew, 1999).

There is little doubt that NPs are key players and potential leaders in the emerging health care system. Although this century brings new opportunities for expanded nursing roles, it also presents challenges for NPs to sustain a holistic perspective in providing care. Intuition has long been acknowledged and reified as a component of complex judgment, understanding, and the perceived view of rational science (Easen & Wilcockson, 1996) as well as a legitimate way of knowing in nursing (Benner, 1984; Benner & Tanner, 1987; Carper, 1978; Rew, 1986, 1989; Young, 1987). In addition, intuition is related to empathy, nursing art, sustained nurse-patient relationships, and holism (Agan, 1987; Rew & Barrow, 1987). According to Rew (2000), intuition, when applied to clinical situations,

> is the act of deciding what to do in a perplexing, often ambiguous and uncertain situations. It is the act of synthesizing empirical, ethical, aesthetic and personal knowledge. Stated another way, intuitive judgment is the decision to act on a sudden awareness of knowledge that is related to previous experience, perceived as a whole, and difficult to articulate. (p. 94)

Whereas the literature addresses numerous barriers to practice from the perspective of scholars and researchers, NPs' perspectives on the problems they confront in everyday practice have not been examined in depth (Martin & Hutchinson, 1999). In addition, the literature is deficient in addressing the role of intuition (i.e., intuitive decision making) by NPs and resultant challenges to maintain holism and caring as the essence of their practices. Therefore, the purpose of this study was to discover, describe, and analyze the stories of novice NPs who use intuitive decision making with clients.

METHOD

The researchers' approach to this study reflects the recognition that multiple research perspectives hold the potential to illuminate the lived experiences of advanced practice nurses (Stevens, 1996). This includes the realization that nursing experiences are socially constructed subjective phenomena and that female nurses' experiences within the patriarchal health care culture may be devalued or ignored (Fonow & Cook, 1991). Interpretive phenomenology is an approach that bridges subjective and objective knowing by focusing on individual perceptions of phenomena and uncovering common themes and universals that emerge from the narratives of persons' lived experiences (Tarzian, 2000). Asking persons to reflect or tell stories of their experiences is empowering; it is also effective in revealing the shared practices and common meanings of those experiences (Brewer & Nelms, 2000). Lowenberg (1993) advocated interpretive research methodology as appropriate for nursing scholarship because this approach emphasizes the importance of everyday life experiences, multiple relativistic constructions of reality, and the incorporation of critical and feminist theory and postmodern perspectives. Therefore, to understand the experiences of NPs who used intuition in clinical decision making with clients, an interpretive phenomenological approach that incorporated critical and feminist theory and postmodern perspectives guided the study.

Participants

Following approval from the authors' Institutional Review Board, the researchers used purposive sampling to solicit the stories of recent graduates of a primary care NP program located within a large metropolitan area in the southeastern United States. Information regarding the purpose and conduct of the study and invitations to voluntarily participate were mailed to NPs who graduated from the program from 1997 to 2000. The researchers received written intentions to participate from several graduates; purposive sampling continued until informational redundancy was reached. A total of 10 NPs participated in the study. Participants averaged 2½ years of experience as

NPs; nine identified their ethnicity as Caucasian and one as African American. The participants' average age was 39 years, and the mean years of experience as registered nurses (RNs) was 13. In the preliminary phase of this study, all participants testified that intuition played an integral role in their practices as expert RNs, that they frequently used and trusted their intuitive decision making within their roles as expert RNs, and that they openly and freely shared their intuitive insights with other nurses and physicians.

Individual, face-to-face interviews were conducted confidentially at a time and place convenient for each participant. To maintain confidentiality and enhance the richness of their stories, participants chose a pseudonym for identification in the study. During the interviews, participants were asked to respond to the following general statement: "Tell me about a time in your experience as an NP when you were aware that intuition was part of your decision making. Share all your thoughts, perceptions, feelings, and actions about the situation until you have no more to say." Using a reflexive dialectic technique, the researcher repeatedly "fed back" the data at several points during each interview for the participant to verify or clarify. Interviews were audiotaped and transcribed verbatim. Transcriptions of the interviews revealed that participants were able to identify and describe numerous clinical interactions with clients when they used intuition as part of their clinical decision making. Following the first-level analysis of the data, participants were mailed a copy of their individual interviews for member checking. According to Guba and Lincoln (1989), member checking involves sharing the results of the findings with participants at multiple levels of the analysis stage and is a critical strategy for verifying data accuracy and credibility.

Data Analysis

The hermeneutic data analysis method developed by Diekelmann and Allen (1989) was used to analyze the transcripts. The procedural steps were as follows: (a) Each text was read individually by the researchers to develop an overall comprehension of the meaning of each interview; (b) the researchers wrote an individual summary of each of the interviews; (c) the researchers met together to discuss their summaries and the meanings embedded in each narrative, and dialogue continued until consensus was reached; (d) the researchers discussed the commonalities and proposed themes that linked common meanings across texts; (e) a constitutive process present in all texts and representing the relationships among themes was identified; and (f) the interpretive analysis was supported using cogent excerpts from the interviews to allow for validation of the findings. In addition, texts were analyzed and examined from critical and feminist theory and postmodern perspectives to situate the stories within their political, social, and cultural contexts.

Methodological rigor was achieved using several strategies included in the trustworthiness criteria (credibility, dependability, confirmability, and transferability) as described by Guba and Lincoln (1989). For example, to enhance credibility, the researchers conducted member checks with participants after the first-level analysis and again at several points during data analysis. Final member checking occurred as participants were asked to review the findings, comment on the fairness and accuracy of interpretations, and confirm descriptions. Credibility was also addressed through peer debriefing; that is, the researchers shared the text summaries, identification of themes, constitutive processes, and final drafts of the findings with a colleague knowledgeable in interpretive phenomenological methods. Because the researchers personally knew the participants as students for 5 to 10 years, they shared a prolonged engagement and persistent observation, which fostered data dependability. Confirmability was approached as each participant verified the data through multiple member-checking opportunities. The researchers believe that transferability of the findings is possible because the sampling was purposive and informational redundancy was achieved. Also, the texts were very rich and deep, and data were congruent across the texts. In addition, one narrative revealed opposing views and different experiences from the other stories and was identified as the "negative case." According to Guba and Lincoln, reporting a negative case experience adds depth to the findings and enhances rigor because these data challenge and then confirm the emerging theory. These multiple cross-checking methods and selective strategies increased methodological rigor and enhanced the trustworthiness of the study.

FINDINGS

All participants began discussing their experiences of using intuition by recalling numerous details of caring for specific clients. Recalling these details was essential for putting voice to their understandings of the role of intuition in their clinical practice as NPs and provided the springboard for uncovering the layers of their experiences. Their stories revealed a process that began with an initial awareness described as "a feeling," which was followed by a series of thoughts and actions that were aptly integrated into the social, political, and temporal contexts of the clinical settings. They completed their stories by sharing how they were able to integrate what they knew, learned, and did in a fashion that enabled them to maintain their sense of integrity, self-esteem, and confidence while caring for themselves and their clients.

The findings of the experiences of these NPs' use of intuition in clinical decision making emerged as a constitutive process that contained the following overlapping themes: (a) reflecting, (b) backing it up, (c) knowing the rules, (d) playing the game, (e) learning lessons, and (f) taking care. These themes are supported using excerpts from participants' interviews in the following discussion.

Theme: Reflecting

Participants began their stories by thinking carefully about previous patient care interactions when they used intuition for clinical decision making. Looking back on these interactions, participants remembered numerous details and a variety of dramatic sensations. Many participants described these sensations negatively, such as "having a very bad feeling," "feeling uncomfortable," or feeling "there was something terribly wrong." They reported having a "nagging sense" about a client's presentation and that there was "something missing" or there was "something they had not done." Following these negative perceptions, some reported visceral reactions, including feeling "twisted inside," "churned up," and "haunted" by certain clients. These feelings were recalled as "automatic," "instant," and "not contrived." Several reported "instantly knowing" about the clients and reported this as similar to having a déjà vu experience. To be sensitive to and aware of these feelings, participants reported that maintaining a "sixth sense" was necessary, as was "always staying open to the nonobvious."

Rose, who worked in a busy prenatal clinic, stated that she tries to "keep an ear open to the unsaid things" and to "stay open so she can pick up on the fuzzy stuff." During a routine prenatal exam, she recalled her feelings about a client and stated, "I had a really bad feeling about this lady. It just struck me. I told the nurses, I think she's going to go bad. Like the kind in [the intensive care unit] that crashes and burns really fast." Pam recalled performing a routine physical examination on a 40-year-old man who made the appointment at the insistence of his wife. He had not had a complete physical examination in many years and was apprehensive about the visit. Because his wife was a friend, Pam, too, felt uncomfortable about doing the prostate examination. She remembered thinking to herself,

> I'll just get in and get out quickly—prostatic exams are not my expertise, and I hadn't done that many. But I had an increased level of suspicion. I felt that something else should be done. I had a strong sense that I should go one step further. So I ordered a PSA [prostate-specific antigen] and referred him to an oncologist. I don't know why I picked up on it. The exam was so fast. It was almost like somebody was standing at my shoulder. Almost like God was whispering at my back. And when the PSA [prostate-specific antigen] came back, it was normal, but the biopsy was malignant.

Theme: Backing It Up

As they became aware of their "gut feelings," participants reported making additional attempts to obtain further objective data to support their instincts. Many "dug deeper and deeper" into the clients' charts, "delved further into their situations," "looked harder and harder for more symptoms," and "asked additional questions" of the clients until they compiled supplementary objective data.

Marion remembered having a nagging feeling that something was not right with a client, which caused her to spend extra time with her. She was persistent and searched back into the patient's old records until she finally found support for her feelings of "not being completely satisfied." She recalled,

> I couldn't put my finger on it, but she just didn't look right. So I went back into her old records. And I finally found that 18 years ago, she had a malignant colectomy, and I thought, oh, so this is what is wrong with this lady! It just kind of hit me. I made the connection, and then I felt satisfied—complete.

Several participants reported attempts to back up their feelings by ordering additional diagnostic tests. Many admitted that if the tests they ultimately wanted to order were not immediately within practice guidelines or insurance protocols, they would build their assessments and diagnoses incrementally until they could justify the specific tests they initially felt were warranted.

Mimi recalled an incident when she garnered the help of office staff members to justify ordering a test for a patient whose insurance would not reimburse payment with her initial diagnosis. She said,

> I had that sinking feeling inside, and instantly I knew that there was not going to be an easy answer for this and that it was ominous. I just knew I had to work her up for cancer. I wanted to get a CEA [carcinoembryonic antigen], but the office staff said, "No, you can't have that." So I said, okay, so we'll draw the CBC [complete blood count] and electrolytes and do all that we can do now. Then, we'll come up with real reasons for going to the next step. Anything I could do to get the evaluation—that's what I wanted. You come up with excuses so that you can get the information that you need.

All participants verified that during the process of intuitive decision making, they were aware that they acknowledged and processed their feelings and then acted on them. As Marion declared, "If you don't act on these feelings, then they are meaningless."

Theme: Knowing the Rules

After responding to their intuitive feelings and taking actions to compile additional data, participants spoke about the importance of having an accurate and substantive knowledge of contextual variables because acting on their intuition felt like "taking a risk." All agreed they needed to be clear of the importance of the information they wanted to share, would "key in on the worst," and would "only share intuitive things of grand or critical importance." Other, less important issues receded into the background.

Comprehensive knowledge of the agency's system and its adherence to protocols was a key factor in the participants' ability to use intuition in clinical decision making. Anna's freedom to use intuition varied greatly in the two settings in which she worked. One setting was a homeless clinic where the clinical guidelines were very general, and the other was a private physician's office whose rules were very structured and rigid. Knowing one's own personality and those of people in charge was also critical—how receptive or open they were for the "soft language." Lynn, who works in a fast-track emergency department (ED), reported that if she has worked extensively with physicians and she perceives them as "receptive," she will tell them,

"I want to learn, so here is my gut feeling—and I will push it. I'll just tell them I have a bad feeling about this, and I will push it." She stated, "The physicians I have worked with a lot—we have a good rapport and they respect me. They are my mentors, and they are the ones I would reveal that inner voice to."

Marion also concurred that one must be aware of the personality of the person in authority. She shared that as an RN, she had worked with a particular physician for a number of years. Now, she works with him and his partner as an NP in their cardiology practice. She recalled,

He trusts my judgment a lot, and he will concur with me. But, the other physician is on the fence about NPs. When it is convenient for him, he is a lot more open and receptive. But he has control issues. He's older and is more old school, and he really doesn't want to hear "that feeling." Some doctors are just not big on intuition.

No matter what the setting, all participants spoke at length about the constraints imposed by time. The amount of time spent with clients was usually specified to a very few minutes, and when they exceed the time allotted, others (particularly physicians) teased or chastised them. As Lynn stated, "After 20 minutes, I came out of the examination room, and they said to me, 'What's the matter, Lynn, we thought we lost you in there.'" Other participants reported suffering more severe repercussions when they spent extra time with clients. They knew that when they exceeded the time allotted, they would have to "catch up" or stay later to complete the examinations of all scheduled clients.

Participants all spoke of the verbal presentation of clients' conditions to physicians as consistently difficult but critically important. They viewed precise communication as a major challenge, one that required conscientious practice, knowledge, and skill very early in their NP careers. They chose language very carefully so that they could be successful at "reporting with bullets of objective data, while trying to get [physicians] to see the big picture." Marion said, "I try to be prepared when I talk to them so I have the important things— because they really don't want to hear 'that feeling.'" Rose confirmed that she was "trained in particulars" and had to be "succinct, to the point, and objective" when presenting clients. She stated that in her setting, they have a "formula of objective data you have to report to the doctors—I have to give them as little information as possible, but I still try to give them the big picture." Participants all reported compiling and practicing as much factual data as possible before communicating with physicians. Anna said that when she prepared to report, she felt like she was "walking on eggs" and that "before starting, you get your ducks in a row."

Theme: Playing the Game

Once participants were confident in the "rules" of the game, they spoke about the next component of the process in ways that simulated "playing the game." They reported recreating the "doctor-nurse game" into a transaction they described with metaphors related to physical movements and images similar to performing a dance or a game. Many stated they would avoid certain physicians who were not receptive to NPs or to "soft language" and would gravitate toward others whom they perceived as more receptive. Tammy stated that it is acceptable to steer away from a protocol as long as she knows the physician is receptive and cooperative. Kimberly, who works with many different physicians in an ED, spoke of how she "tiptoes" around certain physicians and circumvents others. She stated that when she "doesn't feel comfortable about a patient's presentation," she has to know which physician to go to with that information because she has to work with "the flavor of the day." Sometimes, she will wait until physicians "switch shifts and then present the patient to a different physician." She admitted that "this might get me into trouble someday, because it's like a child—if you don't get what you want from one parent, you go to the other." Wanda, Lynn, and Kimberly all admitted they sometimes "avoid presenting [clients] early," obtain more objective data, and "wait for doctors to change shifts" as effective strategies for voicing their concerns, being acknowledged, and receiving the appropriate response.

Some participants chose aggressive metaphors when describing ways they "played the game." During an early experience as an NP, Lynn recalled that she "felt something was very wrong with a client who was in serious pain," and she "played by the rules" by referring the client to a "higher Doc in the main ED." This physician administered intravenous fluids and discharged the client shortly thereafter. The next day, she was admitted to the intensive care unit in acute distress and severe dehydration. Remembering this, Lynn stated,

> I did the right thing. I sought a higher level of care for her [the client], but that did not work out. So the system failed me—my intuition was right, and I did the right thing—but I got burned by the doctor.

When her decisions were overridden, she recalled feeling "pushed back" and "knocked down" by physicians who want to "streamline time in the ED." In a later experience, Lynn spoke of how she again had a bad feeling about a pediatric patient who presented with otitis media but had a suspicious history. This time, however, before referring him on to a "higher" doctor, she "trusted her instinct," obtained more objective data, and waited to present the child to the attending physician. She said,

> I relied on in my intuition, got the chest X ray (which revealed a serious pneumonia), and then went to my attending [physician] for him to see it. It was a no brain-er for him to support me on this one.

Lynn also remembered several instances when she would delay patients in the ED until "shifts changed and new physicians came in" who were "more open and receptive."

Participants all spoke of presenting clients in similar ways and had comparable views of how to play this part of the "game." Telephone reports were identified as particularly difficult and offered special challenges. When Rose reported to a physician by phone, she admitted it was "very difficult to transfer all" she was thinking and feeling over the phone when she could not use her body language to enhance communication. Wanda agreed that she chooses her language very carefully before presenting and recalled many times when she asked herself, "What words can I use to transmit my feelings to this doctor about this patient to help him see why I feel there is something else going on?" Marion stated that "learning how to communicate in a new area with new people—there's an adjustment. You have to choose the right words to get the attention from the right people."

Playing the game included other maneuvers used by participants to obtain the best level of care for clients. Some admitted they detained patients or kept their names on waiting lists so they would be examined again. Others spoke of how they might "exaggerate their [clients'] complaints or length of illness" or "overstate the results of their assessments." Mimi reported that she also taught clients how to play the game when they resisted being referred to the ED for further examination. She recalled,

Patients say to me, "They are not nice to me there—they hassle me." So I just tell the patient what to say. I tell them, when you get to the emergency room, you tell them this and this and this. . . . Then, they will not hassle you, and your insurance will pay.

Rose and Wanda both acknowledged they would send patients on for referral or for admission to a hospital before they have presented the patients' situations to the attending physicians. As Rose stated, "When I'm not comfortable about this patient or I don't get the feedback I want, I just send them in." Mimi affirmed that "the name of the game is taking care of the patient—getting them what they need. If that's what it takes is playing by your rules, then I will play by your rules." Wanda confirmed that "it's a rule game. The bottom line is taking care of the patient while playing by the rules."

Theme: Learning Lessons

Participants reported numerous instances when their intuitive decision making was either validated or blocked by other colleagues. Many spoke of earlier times in their careers when persons with authority agreed or disagreed with them and the lessons they learned as a result. When others involved in their decision making were in agreement, they viewed this as validation, support, and reinforcement of their intuitive decision making. Some of their intuition was met with disagreement, and they recalled this as a negative lesson— one in which they "got burned," "shut down," "knocked down," or "pushed back." Most participants continued to rely on their intuition as a source for decision making, even if earlier attempts had been thwarted. Only one participant, Lucy (whom we identified as the study's negative case), discontinued acting on "gut feelings" after her very first attempt was met with disagreement from a physician. During her first 6 months as an NP, Lucy recalled a time when "deep down inside my intuition told me there was something more going on with this client." She acted on this feeling and referred the client to the physician, who examined and then discharged him. The physician did not admonish Lucy, and she admitted, "He appreciated my concern but discharged him anyway. So I did it once, and it was a gut reaction—but it wasn't validated, so it was wrong." She admitted that she still has intuitive feelings (as she did as an RN for 26 years) but feels "too much like a novice as [an NP]" and does not trust her feelings yet to act on them again.

Shortly after graduating from the NP program, Wanda, Lynn, and Kimberly also had negative experiences when their superiors disagreed with their intuitive decision making. Unlike Lucy, however, they did not abandon their intuitive insights but learned to persist in later situations. They all agreed that persistence was a valuable lesson they learned from earlier experiences and now felt more skilled at persuading physicians to acknowledge their intuition. Wanda recalled a time when a physician initially disagreed with her attempts to follow up with additional testing for a patient but later acquiesced due to her persistence. She recalled,

> I was concerned to the point that if I had not gotten the response I wanted, I had a back up. I was going to follow it through with another physician. But this time, I was met with a positive response—because I was persistent.

Rose agreed that persistence was valuable in pursuing her feelings further with others in authority. She recalled a Friday afternoon when she consulted with the obstetrician on call about a pregnant client whom she had "a really bad feeling about" and was seeking permission to admit the woman to the hospital for observation. After presenting the facts to the on-call physician, she was told to send the client home with instructions for bed rest and a return appointment to the clinic again on Monday. Rose recalled,

> She ended up in the hospital the next day seizing in the waiting room and had a bad DIC [disseminated intravascular coagulation]. I mean, she was really bad. But fortunately, there was a good outcome for her and the baby. And I learned a big lesson that time. I think clinically, I am really sound, but what I learned from it was that I needed to persist. I need to stand my ground when I don't feel good about a patient. When I'm not comfortable, I need to stand up, stand my ground, or just send them in [to the hospital].

Lynn remembered several learning occasions when she acted on her intuitive feelings. During the early months of her career as an emergency room NP, Lynn felt "pushed back" by a physician who discharged a client against her judgment, only to have her return the next day in very serious condition. Recalling this experience, Lynn said,

> I felt frustrated, and I learned that the system failed me—my intuition was right, and I did the right thing. But it did not work out. And it was

very bad, but the thing I learned about that was it was a reinforcement to listen to that voice—and don't not listen to that voice."

In a later situation, Lynn "relied on her intuition" with a pediatric patient and, in this instance, gained support from her attending physician. She said, "So I learned that time that I could come back on board with my intuition and could get some support—even when I was not supported before." She perceived this experience as a relearning to trust her intuition and recalled several subsequent instances when she acted with confidence in her intuitive decision making. She asserted that intuitive decision making is now an everyday occurrence and a natural part of her practice as an NP. She actively tries to "elicit the unspoken word" with clients so she can gain a "personal and intimate view." She declared, "Then I can assess how bad it is. I never turn my head anymore."

Rose agreed that intuitive decision making is "always a general normal day-in, day-out part of my practice, but in some situations, it's consequences are more dramatic." As she reflected on her current practice, she stated,

> I feel personally responsible to stay open to the unsaid things, pick up on the fuzzy stuff, the smaller, more subtle things—because it affects the quality of [clients'] lives for years. And I realize that when I close myself off, I might be missing big opportunities—I might be missing the real reason they are coming in. And I don't like it!

Marion recognized that she routinely reinforces her intuition on an internal level. She described this inner source of knowing as an awareness of being completely satisfied, after which she can "move on to the next thing." She stated that if she did not have this feeling of satisfaction and felt she was "not done," she could not move on. She now "looks for this feeling of satisfaction," which internally provides reinforcement for her intuitive decision making.

Theme: Taking Care

While considering the whole of their experiences of using intuition as NPs, participants identified various techniques as important to taking personal care of themselves and ensuring holistic care of their patients. Participants' caring measures took on diverse forms, but the underlying commonalities centered on specific mental, physical, and psychological self-care activities. These activities promoted participants' satisfaction and well-being and helped them to remain integrated, whole, and caring NPs. They recalled these activities as positive and helpful toward sustaining holism and caring as the essence of their practices. Toward this goal, many stated they shared their paradigm experiences of intuitive decision making with other NPs, whom they viewed as support persons and friends. Some were able to share these experiences with physicians with whom they felt "mutual trust, respect, and confidence." Only Lucy, who was the negative case in this study, stated that after her "gut feeling was wrong" she would not share her intuitive decision making or feelings with anyone.

In taking care of clients, participants reported that they took specific actions to gain further information, provide follow-up, or otherwise achieve closure with clients. Mimi, Rose, and Lynn all confirmed that when they have not had a feeling of completion with clients, they have called the hospitals after hours or on weekends to find out if they were admitted. While working in the ED, Kimberly stated that

> if I don't feel finished with a patient, I leave them on the list and check them later. Or, when I discharge patients who I don't feel should be discharged, I call them at home the next day to make sure they didn't turn blue.

Concerning her self-confidence, she declared,

> I am still in the novice role, and I can't expect others to trust my intuition. But when it is right, I feel justified and know that the next time I have one of those feelings, I will be more assertive.

After receiving validation about their intuitive decision making, participants reported feeling "good," "proud," "excited," "satisfied," and "justified." They all perceived these feelings as positive reinforcement of their intuition and noted that their confidence and assertiveness was enhanced "in order to make a stronger case in the future." Marion remembered feeling "complete and satisfied" with a client and described this as a gratifying situation because she "put all the pieces together and figured it out when several doctors could not." The embodiment of this experience bolstered Marion's confidence in her clinical judgment, reinforced her inner strength, and enhanced her self-esteem.

Many participants confirmed they felt satisfaction and support for their decisions when they knew their intuitive decision making was accurate. Kimberly stated that when her intuitive decision making was "right on the money," she felt "justified" and even "vindicated." Lynn also related the accuracy of her intuition as "reinforcement" and "vindication" for her decision making and actions. They viewed these feelings as positive validation, reinforcement of their clinical judgment, and motivation to hone their intuitive skills for decision making in the future.

Participants recalled the experience of effective intuitive decision making as times when they felt positive about the care they were able to provide for clients. Tammy stated that she felt "okay" about "steering away from the protocols because it was a good decision and it was in the best interests for the patient." Anna recalled feeling "proud and excited" when she intuitively knew the correct diagnosis and treatment for a homeless client. Although expressing sadness when she has to refer clients on to physicians, Mimi admitted that she "goes back and tries to contact a lot of people to find out what has happened to them." She acknowledged that she has a caring connection with many of these clients and is sad about "referring them on" but is proud that she is able to help them within the scope of her rural NP clinic and is convinced she is "providing the best care possible."

Marion also reported that she uses intuition to protect and care for clients. She elaborated on her vigilance and surveillance and admitted she consistently "keys in on the potential for bad things to happen." In safeguarding her clients, she stated, "I always assume the worst and move on to where things don't seem okay. I concentrate my efforts there."

When asked about the possible constraints of clinical guidelines or insurance protocols in providing care for clients, participants discussed various limitations related to the specific settings in which they practiced. However, they acknowledged that when clinical guidelines were somewhat vague and general, they could eventually work with them and obtain the necessary care and follow-up for clients. Wanda asserted, "I never leave the patient high and dry without some other option or treatment or direction to go in. The bottom line is taking care of the patient." Mimi confirmed this commitment with the following statement: "The name of the game is taking care of the patient—making sure the patients get the care that they need."

In this study, participants' narratives began with recollections of initially having various mental, physical, and metaphysical feelings they acknowledged, processed, and acted on. They spoke of these experiences in terms that reflected knowing one's self, the system, and other colleagues within the system. After they gained this knowledge, they spoke of the process of learning to use intuitive decision making in ways that resembled "playing a game." Regardless of whether they were initially successful in playing the game, they learned what behaviors would be effective, or ineffective, in future interactions. Subsequently, their stories revealed a dynamic of experiences that emerged as a constitutive pattern illustrating an iterative process (Polit & Hungler, 1999) of overlapping components. Within this process, the knowledge learned from one component was used as a basis for decision making and moving forward with further activities and alternative methods into the next component. These activities and methods facilitated intuitive decision making for novice NPs as they gained experience and confidence in their new roles. In viewing their narratives, it became evident that participants merged their actions and responses within a progressive reconfiguration of data collection, analysis, interpretation, and decision making. They consciously used this information to weave new findings and insights into their roles as NPs. As their intuitive decision making was repeatedly engaged and validated, their trust and confidence in intuition as a valid way of knowing evolved and grew stronger. Thus, this process was iterative and, with overlapping themes, formed the constitutive pattern of using intuition in clinical decision making with clients (see Figure 1).

IMPLICATIONS

This study reflects the experiences of 10 novice NPs practicing within a southeastern region of the United States. Although the sample was small and homogeneous, the narratives were rich and deep and hold implications for holistic NP practice. The findings of this study support earlier studies of RN practice in which RNs reported the need for validation and reinforcement of intuition as essential for holistic nursing practice (Agan, 1987; Rew, 2000; Young, 1987). Further research of advanced nursing practice is needed that includes a

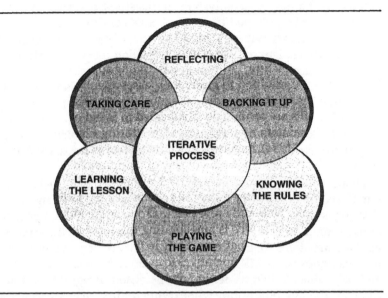

Figure 1:   Constitutive Pattern: An Iterative Process.

larger sample size with diversity of participants and triangulation of methods. Studies of NPs who are more experienced would provide additional information about the role of intuitive decision making in expert NP practice.

The findings must be viewed in light of NP education. NP curricula should include experiences that provide opportunities for students to practice reflective dialogue (Diekelmann, 2001), critical thinking, and intuitive decision making. The results of this study support the notion that these are essential skills for NP graduates and, as such, should be nurtured and role modeled by faculty and clinical preceptors. Given the increased numbers of and responsibilities of NPs in the current and future health care system, the significance of reflective, thoughtful, and intuitive decision making as well as the maximum use of diverse patterns of knowing for nurses cannot be overemphasized (Fawcett, Watson, Neuman, Walker, & Fitzpatrick, 2001).

Additional implications for NP practice can be drawn from these findings. The participants in this study expressed significant concern about working within practice settings that emphasize "objective data only" and "proof by lab values." This was especially evident when they attempted to comprehensively convey clients' conditions to those in charge. Repeatedly, NPs in this study revealed consider-able tension when obliged to report clients' conditions to attending physicians "quickly, with bits of information, while trying to get them to see the whole picture." Although this finding supports the fact that novice NPs use intuition to guide their assessments, obtain further data, and validate that a medical diagnosis exists, it also reflects the notion that NPs are continually challenged to avoid objectifying cli-ents and to maintain a holistic approach during client interactions (Rose & Parker, 1994). Expert NPs, within their own practice settings, may also be struggling with this thorny dilemma and deserve further study.

Finally, RNs encounter numerous challenges while transitioning into the NP role. This study revealed that one of the most significant challenges for novice NPs is ameliorating the requisite transforma-tions in communication patterns. Early in their careers, these partici-pants confronted strong imperatives to modify their previously effec-tive dialogues about clients into "reporting in bullets," "formulas," and "lab values." Their stories reflect a persistent struggle to maintain a holistic nursing philosophy while trying to survive in a system that allows little time or place for personal attention and individualized care. As Lynn stated,

> Here's the dilemma about intuition: As an RN, we are used to relying on it, we trusted it, and doctors respond positively to it. Now, as [an] NP, it is not enough. We have to have a formula for presenting cases to docs, or else we're told "Just forget it—go by the numbers." So much for holism!

This statement supports Hayes (1998), who declared that NP students deserve a quality mentoring experience; it also reinforces the fact that novice NPs must be diligently supported in their efforts to maintain a holistic philosophy and caring center to their nursing practice. For the authors, it conveys a clarion call to NPs, faculty, and members of the profession: It is imperative for all nurses to conscientiously identify and consistently practice activities that enable holistic caring for self, clients, and colleagues.

REFERENCES

Adams, D., & Miller, B. (2001). Professionalism in nursing behaviors of nurse practitioners. *Journal of Professional Nursing, 17*, 203-210.

Agan, R. D. (1987). Intuitive knowing as a dimension of nursing. *Advances in Nursing Science, 10*, 63-70.

Benner, P. (1984). *From novice to expert: Excellence and power in clinical nursing.* Reading, MA: Addison-Wesley.

Benner, P., & Tanner, C. (1987). Clinical judgment: How expert nurses use intuition. *American Journal of Nursing, 87*, 23-31.

Bezyack, M. (1996). Advanced practice: Is it right for you? *The American Journal of Nursing, 96*(15), 17-18.

Brewer, K., & Nelms, T. (2000). A heideggerian hermeneutic study of correctional nurses' experiences of caregiving. *International Journal for Human Caring, 4*, 23-29.

Carper, B. (1978). Fundamental patterns of knowing in nursing. *Advances in Nursing Science, 1*, 13-23.

Diekelmann, N. (2001). Narrative pedagogy: Heideggerian hermeneutical analyses of lived experiences of students, teachers and clinicians. *Advances in Nursing Science, 23*(3), 53-71.

Diekelmann, N., & Allen, D. (1989). A hermeneutic analysis of the NLN criteria for appraisal of baccalaureate programs. In N. Diekelmann, D. Allen, & C. Tanner (Eds.), *The NLN criteria for appraisal of baccalaureate programs: A critical hermeneutic analysis* (pp. 11-34). New York: National League for Nursing.

Easen, P., & Wilcockson, J. (1996). Intuition and rational decision-making in professional thinking: A false dichotomy? *Journal of Advanced Nursing, 24*, 667-673.

Fawcett, J., Watson, J., Neuman, B., Walker, P., & Fitzpatrick, J. (2001). On nursing theories and evidence. *Journal of Nursing Scholarship, 33*, 115-119.

Fonow, M., & Cook, J. (1991). *Beyond methodology: Feminist scholarship as lived research.* Indianapolis: Indiana University Press.

Guba, E., & Lincoln, Y. (1989). *Fourth generation evaluation.* Newbury Park, CA: Sage.

Hayes, E. (1998). Mentoring and self-efficacy for advanced nursing practice: A philosophical approach for nurse practitioner preceptors. *Journal of the American Academy of Nurse Practitioners, 10*(2), 53-57.

Lowenberg, J. (1993). Interpretive research methodology: Broadening the dialogue. *Advances in Nursing Science, 16*(2), 57-69.

Martin, P., & Hutchinson, S. (1999). Negotiating symbolic space: Strategies to increase NP status and value. *The American Journal of Primary Health Care, 22*, 89-102.

Moore, C. (1994). Will the power of the marketplace produce the workforce we need? *Inquiry, 31*, 276-282.

Moser, S., & Armer, J. (2000). NP/MD perceptions of collaborative practice. *Nursing and Health Care Perspectives, 21*, 29-23.

Polit, D., & Hungler, B. (1999). *Nursing research: Principles and methods.* Philadelphia: J. B. Lippincott.

Rew, L. (1986). Intuition: Concept analysis of a group phenomenon. *Advances in Nursing Science, 8*(2), 21-28.

Rew, L. (1989). Intuition in decision-making. *Journal of Nursing Scholarship, 20,* 150-154.

Rew, L. (1999). Unbroken wholeness in advanced practice nursing. *Journal of Holistic Nursing, 17,* 115.

Rew, L. (2000). Acknowledging intuition in clinical decision making. *Journal of Holistic Nursing, 18,* 94-113.

Rew, L., & Barrow, E. (1987). Intuition: A neglected hallmark of nursing knowledge. *Advances in Nursing Science, 10,* 49-62.

Rose, P., & Parker, D. (1994). Nursing: An integration of art and science within the experience of the practitioner. *Journal of Advanced Nursing, 20,* 1004-1010.

Stevens, P. (1996). A critical social reconceptualization of environment in nursing: Implications for methodology. In J. Kenney (Ed.), *Philosophical and theoretical perspectives for advanced nursing practice* (pp. 159-169). Boston: Jones and Bartlett.

Tarzian, A. (2000). Caring for dying patients who have air hunger. *Journal of Nursing Scholarship, 32,* 137-143.

Young, C. (1987). Intuition and nursing process. *Holistic Nursing Practice, 1*(3), 52-62.

Margaret M. Kosowski, R.N., Ph.D., is a professor of nursing at Kennesaw State University in Kennesaw, Georgia. She teaches nursing research, nursing perspectives, and an elective titled "Nursing as Caring." Recent publications are (with Grams, Taylor, & Wilson) "They Took the Time . . . They Started to Care; Stories of African-American Nursing Students in Intercultural Caring Groups" (Advances in Nursing Science, 2001) and (with Grams & Wilson) "Transforming Cultural Boundaries Into Caring Connections" (Journal of Nursing Science, 1997).

Vanice W. Roberts, R.N., D.S.N., is a professor of nursing at Kennesaw State University in Kennesaw, Georgia. She is currently the associate dean for the College of Health and Human Services and the director of the Center for Professional Development and Service in Health Care. She has 27 years of experience in nursing education and nursing administration, with teaching expertise in adult critical care, research, and women's health. Recent publications are "Responding to a Code Blue: Forming Community Partnerships to Help Nurses Return to the Workforce" (Advances for Nurses, 2002) and "Responding to Code Blue: Workforce in Crisis Community Partnerships Returning Nurses to the Workforce," Georgia Nursing, 2001).

EXEMPLAR STUDY 2

Practice Article for Critique

A second article is provided to demonstrate the variety of qualitative methods and to provide the reader the opportunity to critique a qualitative study on his or her own.

Isolation From "Being Alive"

Coping with Severe Nausea and Vomiting of Pregnancy

Beverley O'Brien ▼ Marilyn Evans ▼ Elizabeth White-McDonald

Background: Despite ongoing investigations into specific causes of and treatments for pregnancy-related nausea and vomiting, it remains a common phenomenon of varying intensity that affects the quality of life for both affected women and their families.

Objective: To understand how women cope with severe nausea, vomiting, and/or retching during pregnancy.

Method: Women hospitalized with severe symptoms ($N = 24$) were purposely selected to participate in 24 semistructured interviews and one focus group ($N = 4$).

Results: A process was identified wherein women experienced severe and unrelenting nausea and related symptoms which became progressively more debilitating, leaving them feeling uncertain about when and if they would recover. This caused the women to isolate themselves from their world in an effort to cope with symptoms.

Conclusions: Severe nausea and vomiting of pregnancy is a complex and overwhelming syndrome. Rather than emphasizing a specific treatment for a particular symptom (e.g., vomiting), nurses can intervene to reduce the impact of factors that affect the magnitude of nausea, vomiting, and retching.

Key Words: antenatal comfort • hyperemesis • severe nausea and vomiting of pregnancy

(O'Brien & Naber, 1992; Deuchar, 1995; Koren, 1995; Low, 1996).

Etiological theories and recommendations for appropriate treatment of women with nausea and vomiting of pregnancy have been advanced since antiquity (Fairweather, 1968; O'Brien & Newton, 1991), but many women report that no treatment is consistently helpful (DiIorio, 1985; Mazzotta, Magee, & Koren, 1997; O'Brien & Naber, 1992). Recommendations for nursing care tend to focus on supporting explicit pharmacological and nutritional therapies, rather than supportive emotional care (Aikins-Murphy, 1998; Cowan, 1996; Newman, Fullerton & Anderson, 1993). The investigation of specific etiological and treatment theories rather than the exploration of how affected women actually feel and cope is the focus of most research related to nausea and vomiting of pregnancy (delaRonde, 1994; Aikins-Murphy, 1998; Nelson-Piercy, 1998). The purpose of this investigation was to understand the process through which women cope with their symptoms.

Symptoms that are mild and self-limiting are thought to be "normal" (Deuchar, 1995) and treatment may be deemed unnecessary. This phenomenon has been referred to as "morning sickness" and the etiology of symptoms is generally ascribed to endocrine changes that take place in early pregnancy (Jarnfeldt-Samsioe, Samsioe, & Velinder, 1983; Mori, Amino, Tamaki, Miyai, & Tanizawa, 1988). Mild nausea and vomiting may be "protective" in that a decreased incidence of spontaneous abortion associated with symptoms has been reported (Weigel & Weigel, 1989).

Nausea with or without vomiting or retching in early pregnancy is a common phenomenon affecting 70%–90% of all pregnant women. Symptom severity is highly variable with some women experiencing no nausea, others mild nausea, and yet others relentless nausea along with very frequent vomiting and/or retching. While etiological theories abound, causes for the existence of and variability in symptoms have not been clearly delineated but are thought to be both complex and multifactorial

Beverley O'Brien, DNSc, is Professor, Faculty of Nursing, and Member, Perinatal Research Centre, University of Alberta, Canada.

Marilyn Evans, MN, PhD(c), is Assistant Professor, Brock University, St. Catharines, Ontario, Canada.

Elizabeth White-McDonald, MN, is Clinical Nurse Specialist, Grey Nuns Community Hospital and Health Centre, Edmonton, Alberta, Canada.

Prolonged symptoms that include severe nausea, vomiting, and retching have been referred to as "hyperemesis gravidarum." The definition of hyperemesis gravidarum varies, but generally encompasses women who are deemed sick enough to require hospitalization (Fairweather, 1968; Nelson-Piercy, 1998). Hospitalization is necessitated by nausea, vomiting, and/or retching that result in weight loss (i.e., > 5% of total body weight), electrolyte imbalance, ketosis, and dehydration (American Council of Pharmacy and Chemistry, 1956; Cowan, 1996). Reports on the incidence range from 1% to 3% of all pregnancies and variation in incidence may be due to regional policies governing hospitalization of affected women and true demographic differences (Nelson-Piercy, 1998; Fairweather, 1968; Klebanoff, Koslowe, Kaslow, & Rhoads, 1985). Prior to the introduction of intravenous fluids, a maternal death rate was recorded in many countries as a result of severe dehydration and ketosis (Fairweather, 1968; O'Brien & Newton, 1991). While maternal death is now rare, more severe symptoms are likely to continue for longer (Zhou, O'Brien, & Relyea, 1999) and symptoms that continue into the third trimester are associated with a higher incidence of low birth weight infants (Gross, Librach, & Cecutti, 1989; Weigel & Weigel, 1989). In a Canadian study, 3,201 women with nausea and vomiting were surveyed to assess psychosocial morbidity associated with varying degrees of nausea and vomiting. They reported that they felt depressed and their interpersonal relationships were adversely affected. Some desired therapeutic abortion to alleviate their symptoms (Mazzotta, Magee, & Koren, 1997). In a prospective British study of 266 women, Gadsby (1994) reported that of 206 women employed outside the home, 73 missed work for an average of 22 hours each, thus demonstrating the significant economic impact of severe symptoms.

The caregiver's perspective of hospitalization with severe nausea and vomiting may differ significantly from a woman's experience. There is great variability in an individual's ability to describe a subjective sensation (Lenz, Pugh, Milligan, Gift, & Suppe, 1997). Factors other than nausea and vomiting and/or retching may be an integral part of the experience. For example, O'Brien and Naber (1992) reported that maternal guilt is frequently associated with accepting pharmaceutical therapy because of potential adverse effects on fetal development. Most women in this study reported mild-to-moderate symptoms. Strategies for appropriate care may be more evident if nurses gain insight into how women cope with nausea and vomiting that is severe enough to require hospitalization.

The purpose of this study is to understand how women cope with severe pregnancy-related nausea and vomiting and/or retching. Symbolic interactionism is an approach to the scientific study of how humans conduct themselves in their natural settings and within their social groupings (Blumer, 1969, p. 47). "The researcher needs to understand behavior as the participants understand it, learn about their world, learn their interpretation of self in the interaction, and share their definitions" (Chenitz & Swanson, 1986, p. 7). This theoretical approach is appropriate when ascribing meaning to a dynamic event (Wuest, 1995), such as nausea and vomiting or retching, in that the goal is an understanding of the process through which those experiencing its most severe manifestations are able to cope.

Methods

Sample Selection

Pregnant women admitted to a large tertiary care hospital in western Canada because of severe nausea, vomiting, or retching were eligible for inclusion. Following approval by appropriate ethics committees, the unit coordinator approached eligible women to ascertain whether or not they would be interested in meeting with a member of the research group to learn more about the study.

A total of 24 women participated in the study. Of these, 16 women took part in one interview, 4 women took part in two interviews, and 4 took part in a focus group. Interviews lasted 45 to 90 minutes, and 21 took place while the participant was hospitalized (i.e., one participant was interviewed on two occasions while hospitalized). One was interviewed a second time by telephone following discharge; and two were interviewed during home visits, one after her birth and one after her abortion. After data were analyzed, 4 women who had been hospitalized but had not previously taken part in the study were asked to describe their experience in a focus group (lasting 2 hours); they were then presented with study findings and asked to comment. Two of the women were still experiencing symptoms at 34 and 36 weeks' gestation, respectively. The other two had given birth in the past 4 to 6 weeks.

Women taking part in the study ranged in age from 18 to 41 years. This was the first pregnancy for 8 of the women, the second for 15, and the third for 1. While most of the women were White, they came from a variety of cultural backgrounds (i.e., Caribbean [1], Aboriginal [2], and Asian [1]). All but two were high school graduates; 10 had postsecondary and three had postgraduate educational backgrounds.

Instruments and Procedures

A descriptive-exploratory study was conducted using grounded theory procedures and techniques described by Strauss and Corbin (1990). Data were collected through individual interviews with symptomatic hospitalized women and analysis was concurrent with data collection. Initially, the sample was one of convenience with hospitalized volunteers being asked to describe how they coped with their experience. This was done in a private area, often at the bedside. Sampling became more purposive as categories began to emerge and as the research group for-

> Nausea in early pregnancy is a common phenomenon

mulated specific questions. Some participants were interviewed a second time during or immediately following their pregnancy so that existing codes and developing categories could be further clarified. The emerging theory was presented to a focus group of affected women for comment, confirmation, and clarification because it was judged that findings would be relevant only if these women recognized their own experience in the presented description. All that was said in the interviews and focus group was tape recorded and transcribed verbatim.

The interview format was semi-structured with general questions being posed and prompters used when necessary (e.g., "What is it like to be in hospital when you are feeling this sick? What have those close to you, your employer, and your caregivers, done that has been helpful or not helpful? What makes you feel better or worse?"). The research group met regularly while planning the study and throughout the data collection and analysis period. The two members of the group who interviewed participants underwent a training period, which included role playing during videotaped practice sessions so that they could refine their interviewing skills. Although neither of the interviewers provided direct care to participants in the study, both were experienced maternity nurses who were sensitive to indications that symptoms were worsening. If this happened, the interview was stopped and rescheduled for a time when the participant was feeling better.

The analytic strategy for the analysis included open coding or line-by-line examination of all transcriptions as well as interviewer notes. Coding involved the implementation of controls and procedures, stated a priori, to analyze data so that an objective and systematic approach was assured. Coding comprises examining, comparing, conceptualizing, and categorizing data (Strauss & Corbin, 1990). Each interview was read, reread, and coded by at least two of the four members of the research group. Lines, paragraphs, and words were coded to represent categories in the discussion. Emerging categories were discussed and final categories were determined by consensus within the research group. Data were then reconstructed by linking categories and subcategories within a set of relationships so that the context in which the experience occurred could be described (axial coding). A concept (i.e., core category) around which all emerging categories could be related was selected. The emerging theory was refined and confirmability was assessed by both research group consensus and the response of the focus group members.

Results

A basic social process was identified wherein women experienced severe and unrelenting nausea, vomiting, and related symptoms which began insidiously very early in pregnancy and became progressively more debilitating, leaving them feeling uncertain about ever feeling "normal" again. The women engaged in a "struggle" with the profound changes that were occurring within their bodies, which they personified and believed were capable of annihilating them. They had difficulty communicating the impact of these changes to those whom they relied on for support. The women increasingly withdrew from all aspects of daily living so that they could cope, which left them feeling isolated from all aspects of their lives.

The core category was the process of increasingly complete physical, social, and emotional isolation to cope with unrelenting and severe symptoms. This process and finally its resolution was characterized by five stages, which were labeled: (a) rationalization, (b) recognition (internal and external), (c) domination, (d) annihilation, and (e) renewal (Figure 1). The first stage did not occur or occurred only briefly in women who had previously experienced severe symptoms. When all stages occurred, they occurred sequentially. Tensions experienced by the participants were evident throughout all but the final stage of the process and included feelings of (a) profound loneliness coexisting with a need for almost complete social and physical withdrawal, (b) loss of control over self and virtually every aspect of living coexisting with a need for recognition and support to cope with symptoms, and (c) guilt while immersed in feelings of helplessness.

> *Increasing isolation was associated with unrelenting nausea, incessant vomiting, and retching*

▼▼▼

Stages in the Process of Increasing Isolation With Unrelenting Nausea, Vomiting, and Retching

Rationalization. Women who did not experience severe symptoms during a previous pregnancy interpreted early symptoms as a transient phenomenon that would have minimal impact on their usual functioning. For many, nausea was expected and deemed to be a normal event. Some were even reassured by the presence of early nausea because they felt this confirmed their pregnancy. Others rationalized their symptoms as being due to something they ate, or the "flu."

The women created a balance between identifying sources of support to help them deal with their symptoms and maintaining their preconception levels of functioning. They expect that nausea and related symptoms would resolve quickly without any particular intervention and they would resume activities that they were engaged in prior to conception. Their initial withdrawal and subsequent isolation from usual activities was expected to be temporary. One woman said, "I just woke up one morning and it was there. I thought it is probably just something I ate the previous night and I thought, 'This is going to pass.' The problem was, it never passed." Another woman noted, "I kept saying, 'Tomorrow I'll feel good. Tomorrow I'll feel good, and it just never happened'."

Recognition (Internal and External). As women moved into the next stage, they recognized that strategies to relieve the "flu" were not working. They were keenly aware of the pervasiveness and severity of their symptoms (i.e., internal

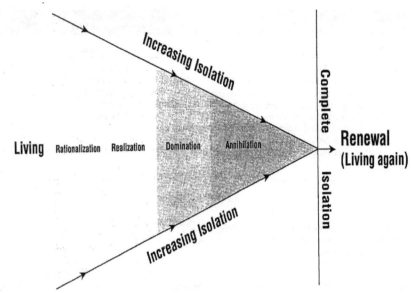

FIGURE 1. Isolated from living: process of coping with severe nausea, vomiting, and/or retching of pregnancy.

recognition) before those around them accepted that they were not well. They reported numerous related physiological, psychological, and situational dimensions to describe how they were feeling (Table 1). They began to feel uncertain about if and when symptoms would end and viewed themselves as being "sick." They coped by isolating themselves from usual contacts in order to minimize the embarrassment of being "caught vomiting," the frustration of others dismissing their symptoms, and ongoing fatigue. One woman noted, "I've had severe flu where I've been throwing up and got so shaky; but you only have one day like that, then you start your recovery...and there was no end to this." Another reported, "I know that people get morning sickness, but this is excessive; people would say 'it's quite normal' and I don't know if that was helpful or not because for me it felt excessive."

External recognition is the informal and formal response of others to the increasing isolation of affected women and to what they believe these women are experiencing. External recognition may or may not be helpful. Informal external recognition comes from spouses, other family members, friends, and coworkers. One woman reported,

> My husband has gone through this with me already. "What do you mean you are too sick to go to work? You did in your first pregnancy. Come on, you can't be that much worse." And he's a nice guy! I said, "I hate you! Can't you understand what I'm feeling?" And then finally, when I was admitted to the hospital, he said, "You're really sick, aren't you?" ...and now he's really good about it, but he's tired of it, too.

Another said, "The people at work don't understand this being sick. They think I'm probably making it up"

while another said, "I am at the point where my family is tired of it...and there is no end in sight".

Formal recognition comes from healthcare professionals and employers. As indicated in a previous quote, being admitted to the hospital is an important source of formal recognition. Women did not believe that their employers and health professionals recognized or understood what they were going through. They appreciated nurses who offered support by asking how they were feeling and listening to them. Others reported that healthcare professionals either doubted their symptoms or thought they were trivial. One woman said, "I just hate that it is downplayed. When you are feeling sick and want somebody to help you, it is hard to ask for that help when you know it is going to come back to you, 'oh, all you need to do is sleep it off.'" A single teen reported, "I felt that because I was not in labor that it wasn't important. I was really sick and feeling crappy and I didn't understand why I was kind of just put into a corner...and I just didn't feel like it [severe nausea and vomiting] was important." Another woman said, "If one more person says to me, 'Here, have a cracker,' or 'Maybe you should drink some ginger ale,' I am going to bop them. I found that nothing helped for the first six months." The women were grateful when nurses and other caregivers indicated that they recognized and understood their need to isolate themselves.

Domination. Symptoms dominated severely affected women who also reported pervasive feelings of fear, guilt, and loss of control. As one participant said, "It seems to have a life of its own." Another reported,

> All you think about is how you are feeling. You don't think about what you are going to do with your child. You are just thinking about feeling sick...it doesn't ever all go away. There is never a

---

TABLE 1. Dimensions of Severe Nausea and Vomiting of Pregnancy

Physiological	Psychological	Situational
Unrelenting...	Feelings of...	Intolerance of...
Nausea, vomiting, retching of stomach acid and bile	Profound aloneness	Odors
Anorexia, hunger, weight loss, ptylism, alterations in taste	Embarrassment	Loud noises
(e.g., weird, metallic, yukky); heartburn, gastric pain,	Humiliation	Lights
"heavy," weakness; fatigue; sleepiness; tremors	Helplessness	Movement
(i.e., shakiness); pallor; oliguria; diarrhea; dryness of	Guilt	Withdrawal from...
mouth, skin; alopecia; flu-like symptoms including	Being overwhelmed	Employers and colleagues
dizziness, lightheadedness, headache, arthralgia	Being consumed	Friends
		Family
		Self

---

time when you're walking around thinking, 'Jeez, I don't feel like throwing up right now?'... It sort of takes priority over anything else.

The domination affects their entire being as exemplified by one woman, who said, "I became more mechanical. Everything I did was on a schedule and if I stuck to that schedule, I knew I could make it to the end of the day. Just get to that point where I knew I could sit on the couch...and that is how I lived." Another said, "So it has been pretty bad...it just takes a toll on your family, your mental being, your physical being, marriage, everything."

Annihilation. Participants believed that they were completely alone (i.e., physically, emotionally, and socially isolated from being alive) and started to fear a partial or total loss of self. To illustrate their feelings of loss, all women tended to make remarkably similar statements suggesting that they were isolated from being alive. The statements included comments such as, "I want my life back; I am dying; I felt really not alive. It's almost like I really don't exist anymore, and I am hyperemesis." One woman said, "I felt like I was in the twilight zone. I really did. I've never felt like that before, even when my mother died. It is a horrible experience when your mother dies, and she died of cancer so it was a long drawn out thing but you can still live." Two of the women elected to have therapeutic abortions and others fantasized about having a miscarriage or considered having an abortion. One woman said, "It was so bad I was even thinking about getting an abortion because I couldn't endure it anymore...I thought this is not worth killing myself over."

Renewal. Symptoms subsided and for some women this occurred slowly over the course of the pregnancy or when the pregnancy ended. For others, the symptoms subsided around 16 to 22 weeks gestation. Participants were relieved when they started to "feel alive" and recognize themselves in ways that they had taken for granted prior to becoming pregnant. One woman noted that the week after her abortion was, "...one of the best weeks of my life because I was able to sit on the deck and the weather was warm and I could read my book and I was in the park and went for walks and I was

alive!" While the stages were sequential, associated tensions were evident throughout all stages of the process.

Tensions Evident Throughout the Process

Loneliness Versus Need for Social and Physical Withdrawal. The most pervasive feelings were those of profound loneliness coexisting with the need for isolation that necessitated social and physical withdrawal. The women experienced a profound sense of loneliness even while craving privacy. For example,

It is a kind of loneliness. You look around and you see all these other women with babies and you know there are smiles on their faces. I couldn't even stand for anyone to be in the room, I was just so sick that [I] just wanted to pull a blanket over [my] head...

Another said, "It's kind of a lonely experience, it's very lonely." One noted, "What helped me is saying that I am not the only one." Much of the increased isolation stemmed from disbelief by others that their symptoms were severe. One woman said, "[This is] so hard because everyone is so different. The majority of people aren't this sick during their pregnancy or it stops." Another said, "[Most say], 'it's no big deal, everybody has morning sickness,' but when it is all the time, it is hard to keep going while people say, 'ignore it and it will go away' but it doesn't. I think it is hard that people look at me and say, 'Well, everybody has babies.'"

Loss of Personal Control Versus Need for Support From Others. Women also feared losing control over self and every aspect of living while feeling a desperate need for recognition and support so that they could cope with symptoms and assure self survival. Included was a loss of control of self (public vomiting), family (unable to care for children), and occupation (unable to function at preconception level). Affected women felt that they were surrendering to or being controlled by their symptoms. One woman said, "I couldn't eat and I thought, well, that's stupid. I should be able to eat but I can't. I thought they [caregivers] must think that I am crazy or something if I am not able to eat."

Guilt Versus Helplessness. They experienced feelings of guilt associated with not being able to fulfill their preconception roles, harming the anticipated baby, and somehow being responsible for the severity of their own symptoms, all the while being immersed in feelings of helplessness. The isolation can be complete in that the women felt physically as well as emotionally and socially isolated. Interaction with others was tiring and even embarrassing since many feared public vomiting. For example, one woman noted that she did not want others to know she was vomiting, "Even at home, I'll run into the bathroom and lock the door. I'll even run the water while I'm doing it." Another said, "I'm afraid to go anywhere because I don't want to be out in public and throwing up. So I just don't go anywhere. I stay at home and it's between my bed and my rocking chair and the toilet and that's basically what my life consists of."

Several women felt emotionally isolated because they believed they had done something to precipitate their symptoms. Feelings of "Being Different" led to guilt and increasing isolation. These feelings caused fear of possessing physical or psychiatric qualities that would harm the developing embryo. One woman said, "[I felt] sad and like a failure because I was back in the hospital. I thought there was something more that I could have done. Even though I know I couldn't have done more than what I did, but..." Another reported, "I'm always telling my husband, 'We can't do that because I'm not feeling good.' [I am telling] my little boy, 'I can't play with you right now because I am not feeling good enough.' I always feel like I'm disappointing people all the time."

Discussion

Participants reported a process that involved increasing levels of social, emotional, and physical isolation that culminated with feelings of "not being alive." Increasing isolation was associated with unrelenting nausea, incessant vomiting, and retching, and a myriad of associated symptoms and feelings as well as an inability to communicate the depth of the experience to those on whom they relied for support.

It is reasonable to hypothesize that if symptom severity can be diminished, the degree of isolation required to cope might be attenuated. Existing symptom theories were assessed to further understand the nature of appropriate support for those experiencing unpleasant symptoms. The middle range theory of unpleasant symptoms was developed to provide a vehicle for integrating information about a variety of symptoms, including nausea (Lenz, Pugh, Milligan, Gift, & Suppe, 1997). The utility of the theory is that it can explain and guide research and practice associated with an array of unpleasant symptoms; some symptoms may precipitate others or several symptoms may occur simultaneously. Thus, interventions may be introduced to treat less recalcitrant symptoms associated with severe nausea and vomiting. Lenz and associates (1996) posit that physical, emotional, and situational factors interact causing a synergistic effect that affects intensity, duration, distress, and timing of unpleasant symptoms, which most often are experienced simultaneously. Rather than emphasizing a specific treatment for a particular symptom (e.g.,

vomiting), nurses can intervene to reduce the impact of predisposing and coexisting factors that affect the magnitude of nausea, vomiting, retching, and other symptoms. More definitive guidelines are an important area for future clinical research .☑

Accepted for publication April 2, 2002.
The authors thank research assistants Joan Bowman, RN; Annita Damsma MN; and Rhonda Harris, MN; for their work on this study.
Corresponding author: Beverley O'Brien, DNSc, Faculty of Nursing, 3rd Floor Clinical Sciences Building, Edmonton, Alberta, Canada, T6G 2G3 (e-mail: Beverley.obrien@ualberta.ca).

References

Aikins-Murphy, P. (1998). Alternative therapies for nausea and vomiting of pregnancy. *Obstetrics & Gynecology, 91,* (1), 149-155.

Blumer, H. (1969). *Symbolic interactionism: Perspective and method.* Prentice-Hall Inc., New Jersey.

Cowan, M. J. (1996). Hyperemesis gravidarum: Implications for home care and infusion therapies. *Journal of Intravenous Nursing, 19* (1), 46-58.

delaRonde, S. K. (1994). Nausea and vomiting in pregnancy. *Journal of the Society of Obstetrics & Gynecology, 16,* 2035-2041.

Chenitz W. C. & Swanson, J. M. (1986). *From practice to grounded theory: Qualitative research in nursing.* Menlo Park, CA: Addison-Wesley, p 7.

Deuchar, N. (1995). Nausea and vomiting in pregnancy: A review of the problem with particular regard to psychological and social aspects. *British Journal of Obstetrics & Gynecology, 102,* 6-8.

Dilorio, C. (1985). First trimester nausea in pregnant teenagers: Incidence, characteristics, intervention. *Nursing Research, 34,* 372-377.

Fairweather, D. V. I. (1968). Nausea and vomiting in pregnancy. *American Journal of Obstetrics & Gynecology, 102,* 135-175.

Gross, S., Librach, C., & Cecutti, A. (1989). Maternal weight loss associated with hyperemesis gravidarum: A predictor of fetal outcome. *American Journal of Obstetrics & Gynecology, 160,* 906-909.

Iatrakis, G. M., Sakellaropoulos, G. G., Kourkoubas, A. H., & Kabounia, S. E. (1988). Vomiting and nausea in the first 12 weeks of pregnancy. *Psychotherapy and Psychosomatics, 49,* 22-24.

Jarnfelt-Samsioe, A., Samsioe, G., & Velinder, G. (1983). Nausea and vomiting in pregnancy—A contribution to its epidemiology. *Gynecological & Obstetrical Investigation, 16,* 221-229.

Koren, G. (1995). Drug of choice for morning sickness. *Canadian Family Physician, 41,* 1671-1674.

Lenz, E., Pugh, L., Milligan, R., Gift, A., Suppe. F. (1997). The middle-range theory of unpleasant symptoms: An update. *Advances in Nursing Science, 19*(3); 14-27.

Low, K. G. (1996). Nausea and vomiting in pregnancy: A review of the research. *Journal of Gender, Culture & Health, 1* (3), 151-172.

Mazzotta, P., Magee, L., & Koren, G. (1997). Therapeutic abortions due to severe morning sickness: An unacceptable combination. *Canadian Family Physician, 43,* 1055-7.

Mori, M., Amino, N., Tamaki, H. Miyai, K., & Tanizawa, O. (1988). Morning sickness and thyroid function in normal pregnancy. *Obstetrics & Gynecology, 72,* 355-358.

Nelson-Piercy, C. (1998). Treatment of nausea and vomiting in pregnancy: When should it be treated and what can be safely taken? *Drug Safety, 19* (2), 155-164.

Newman, V, Fullerton, J. T. & Anderson, P. O. (1993). Clinical advances in the management of severe nausea and vomiting during pregnancy. *Journal of Obstetrical, Gynecological & Neonatal Nursing, 22* (6), 483-490.

O'Brien, B. & Naber, S. (1992). Nausea and vomiting during pregnancy: Effects on the quality of women's lives. *Birth, 19* (3), 138-143.

O'Brien, B. & Newton, N. (1991). Psyche vs. Soma : Historical beliefs about nausea and vomiting during pregnancy. *Journal of Psychosomatic Obstetrics & Gynecology, 12,* 91-120.

Weigel, M & Weigel, R. (1989). Nausea and vomiting of early pregnancy and pregnancy outcome. A meta-analytical review. *British Journal of Obstetrics and Gynaecology, 96,* 1312-1318.

Wuest, J. (1995). Feminist grounded theory: An exploration of the congruency and tensions between two traditions in knowledge discovery. *Qualitative Health Research, 5*(1), 125-137.

Zhou, Q., O'Brien, B., & Relyea, J. (1999). Severity of nausea and vomiting during pregnancy: What does it predict? *Birth, 26,* 108-114.

References and Bibliography

Abbott, P. (2000). The challenges of data mining in large nursing home datasets. In V. Saba, R. Carr, W. Sermeus, & P. Rocha (Eds.), *Nursing informatics 2000: One step beyond: Evolution of technology and nursing* (pp. 53–60). New Zealand: Adis.

Allen, M., et al. (2002). *Essential nursing references.* Retrieved October 28, 2003, from http://www.nin.org/ninjournal/nursingreferences.htm

Alvesson, M., & Sköldberg, K. (2000). *Reflexive methodology new vistas for qualitative research.* London: Sage.

Babbie, E. (1990). *Survey research methods* (pp. 65–117). Belmont, CA: Wadsworth.

Bakken, S. (2001). An informatics infrastructure for evidence-based practice. *Journal of the American Medical Informatics Association, 8*(3), 199–201.

Blalock, H. (1969). *Theory construction.* Englewood Cliffs, NJ: Prentice-Hall.

BMJ Publishing Group Ltd. *Evidence based nursing.* Retrieved September 10, 2003, from http://ebn.bmjjournals.com/.

Bryman, A., & Burgess, R. (Eds.). (1999). *Qualitative Research Vols. I, II, III, IV.* Thousand Oaks, CA: Sage Publications.

Burns, N. (1989). Standards for qualitative research. *Nursing Science Quarterly, 2*(1), 44–52.

Burns, N., & Grove, S. K. (1997). *The practice of nursing research* (3rd ed.). Philadelphia: Saunders.

Chinn, P., & Kramer, M. (1999). *Theory and nursing: A systematic approach* (5th ed.). St. Louis, MO: Mosby.

Chinn, P. L., & Jacobs, M. K. (1999). *Theory and nursing.* St. Louis, MO: Mosby.

Cochrane Collaboration, The. (2003). *The Cochrane collaboration.* Retrieved September 11, 2003, from http://www.cochrane.org/.

Cohen, J. (1988). *Statistical power analysis for the behavioral sciences* (2nd ed.). Hillsdale, NJ: Erlbaum.

Crabtree, B., & Miller, W. (Eds.). (1992). *Doing qualitative research.* Newbury Park, CA: Sage.

Creswell, J. (1998). *Qualitative inquiry and research design choosing among five traditions.* Thousand Oaks, CA: Sage.

Delaney, C., Ruiz, M., Clarke, M., & Srinivasan, P. (2000). Knowledge discovery in database: Data mining NMDS. In V. Saba, R. Carr, W. Sermeus, & P. Rocha (Eds.), *Nursing informatics 2000: One step beyond: Evolution of technology and nursing* (pp. 61–65). New Zealand: Adis.

139

Denzin, N., & Lincoln, Y. (Eds.). (2000). *Handbook of qualitative research* (2nd ed.). Thousand Oaks, CA: Sage.

Dey, I. (1999). *Grounding grounded theory guidelines for qualitative research.* San Diego, CA: Academic Press.

Devellis, R. F. (1991). *Scale development: Theory and applications.* Newbury Park, CA: Sage.

DiCenso, A., Cullum, N., & Ciliska, D. (1998). Implementation forum. Implementing evidence-based nursing: Some misconceptions. *Evidence-Based Nursing, 1*(2), 38–40.

Dillman, D. (1999). *Mail and internet surveys* (2nd ed.). New York: Wiley.

Dubin, R. (1969). *Theory building.* New York: Free Press.

Edgerton, S. (1988). *Guide to critique of philosophical research.* Unpublished manuscript, Steinhardt School of Education, New York University.

Edward G. Miner Library, University of Rochester Medical Center. (2003). *Evidence-based filters for ovid CINAHL.* Retrieved September 11, 2003, from http://www.urmc.rochester.edu/hslt/miner/digital_library/tip_sheets/Cinahl_eb_filters.pdf

Ely, M., Anzul, M., Friedman, T., Garner, D., & Steinmetz, A. (1991). *Doing qualitative research: Circles within circles.* New York: Falmer.

Fawcett, J. (1993). *Analysis and evaluation of nursing theories.* Philadelphia: Davis.

Fawcett, J. (1995). *Analysis and evaluation of conceptual models of nursing.* Philadelphia: Davis.

Fawcett, J. (1999). *The relationship of theory and research.* Philadelphia: Davis.

Fink, A. (1995). *How to sample in surveys.* Thousand Oaks, CA: Sage.

Fitzpatrick, J., & Whall, A. (1996). *Conceptual models of nursing analysis and application.* Stamford, CT: Appleton & Lang.

Geitgey, & Metz. (1973). In F. Downs & M. Newman (Eds.), *A source book of nursing research.* Philadelphia: Davis.

George, J. (2002). *Nursing theories: The base for professional practice.* Upper Saddle, NJ: Pearson Education Inc. Appleton & Lang.

Gergen, M., & Gergen, K. (2000). Qualitative inquiry. In N. Denzin & Y. Lincoln (Eds.), *Handbook of qualitative research* (2nd ed.). Thousand Oaks, CA: Sage.

Giacquinta, J., Bauer, J., & Levin, J. (1993). *Beyond technology's promise.* New York: Cambridge University Press.

Given, B., & Given, C. W. (1992). Patient and family caregiver reaction to new and recurrent breast cancer. *Journal of the American Medical Women's Association, 47*(5), 201–206.

Goodwin, L. K., Iannachione, M., & Hammond, W. (2000). Data mining methodology for outcomes analysis in complex clinical problems. In V. Saba, R. Carr, W. Sermeus, & P. Rocha (Eds.), *Nursing informatics 2000: One step beyond: Evolution of technology and nursing* (pp. 66–72). New Zealand: Adis.

Groves, R., Dillman, D., Eitinge, J., & Little, R. (2001). *Survey nonresponse.* New York: Wiley.

HealthWeb. (2002). *Electronic discussion groups for nursing.* Retrieved October 14, 2003, from http://healthweb.org/browse.cfm?categoryid=1723

Henry, G. (1990). *Practical sampling.* Thousand Oaks, CA: Sage.

Hoskins, C. N. (1980). Psychometrics in nursing research: Construction of an interpersonal conflict scale. *Research in Nursing and Health, 4,* 243–249.

Hoskins, C. N. (1988). *The Partner Relationship Inventory.* Palo Alto, CA: Consulting Psychologists Press.

Kim, J., & Mueller, C. W. (1978a). *Factor analysis: Statistical methods and practical issues.* Beverly Hills, CA: Sage.

Kim, J., & Mueller, C. W. (1978b). *Introduction to factor analysis: What it is and how to do it.* Beverly Hills, CA: Sage.

Kish, L. (1965). *Survey sampling.* New York: Wiley.

Kuzel, A. (1992). Sampling in qualitative inquiry. In B. Crabtree & W. Miller (Eds.), *Doing qualitative research.* Newbury Park, CA: Sage.

Light, R. J., Singer, J. D., & Willett, J. B. (1990). *By design* (pp. 186–210). Cambridge, MA: Harvard University Press.

Lincoln, Y. S., & Guba, E. G. (1985). *Naturalistic inquiry.* Beverly Hills, CA: Sage.

Locke, H. J., & Wallace, K. M. (1959). Short marital adjustment and prediction tests: Their reliability and validity. *Marriage and Family Living, 21,* 251–255.

Lofland, J., & Lofland, L. H. (1984). *Analyzing social settings: A guide to qualitative observation and analysis* (2nd ed.). Belmont, CA: Wadsworth.

Lohr, S. (1999). *Sampling design and analysis.* Belmont, CA: Wadsworth.

Manchester, P. (1986). Analytic philosophy and foundational inquiry: The method. In P. Munhall & C. Oiler, *Nursing research: A qualitative perspective* (pp. 229–249). Norwalk, CT: Appleton-Century-Crofts.

Mangione, T. (1995). *Mail surveys* (pp. 38–87). Thousand Oaks, CA: Sage.

Mariano, C. (1990). Qualitative research: Instructional strategies and curricular considerations. *Nursing and Health Care, 11*(7), 354–359.

Mariano, C. (1995). The qualitative research process. In L. Talbot (Ed.), *Principles and practices of nursing research.* St. Louis, MO: Mosby.

Marriner-Tomey, A. (1994). *Nursing theorists and their work.* St. Louis, MO: Mosby.

Mathews, V. D., & Mihanovich, C. S. (1963). New orientations on marital maladjustment. *Marriage and Family Living, 25,* 300–304.

Miles, M. B., & Huberman, A. M. (1994). *Qualitative data analysis: A sourcebook of new methods.* Beverly Hills, CA: Sage.

Morse, J. (Ed.). (1994). *Critical issues in qualitative research methods.* Thousand Oaks, CA: Sage.

Munhall, P. (2001). *Nursing research: A qualitative perspective* (3rd ed.). Sudbury, MA: Jones & Bartlett Publishers and National League for Nursing.

Nicoll, L. (Ed.). (1997). *Perspectives on nursing theory.* Philadelphia: Lippincott.

Nunnally, J., & Bernstein, J. H. (1994). *Psychometric theory* (3rd ed.). New York: McGraw-Hill.

Patton, M. (1990). *Qualitative evaluation and research methods* (2nd ed.). Newbury Park, CA: Sage.

Pedhazur, E. J., & Schmelkin, L. P. (1991). *Measurement, design, and analysis: An integrated approach.* Hillsdale, NJ: Erlbaum.

Perloff, E., Director. (1996). Health and Psychosocial Instruments [CD-ROM]. Pittsburgh, PA: Behavioral Measurement Database Services.

Polit, D. R., & Hungler, B. P. (1999). *Nursing research. Principles and methods* (7th ed.). New York: Lippincott.

Scheaffer, R. (1996). *Elementary survey sampling.* Belmont, CA: Wadsworth.

Slonim, M. (1960). *Sampling.* New York: Simon & Schuster.

Spector, P. E. (1992). *Summated rating scale construction.* Newbury Park, CA: Sage.

Strauss, A. L., & Corbin, J. (1998). *Basics of qualitative research: Techniques and procedures for developing grounded theory* (2nd ed.). Thousand Oaks, CA: Sage.

Tabachnick, B. G., & Fidell, L. S. (1989). *Using multivariate statistics.* New York: HarperCollins.

Tesch, R. (1990). *Qualitative research: Analysis types and software tools.* Bristol, PA: Falmer.

Walker, L., & Avant, K. (1983). *Strategies for theory construction in nursing.* Norwalk, CT: Appleton-Century-Crofts.

Waltz, C., & Bausell, R. B. (1981). *Nursing research: Design, statistics and computer analysis.* Philadelphia: Davis.

Weitzman, E. (2000). Software and qualitative research. In N. Denzin & Y. Lincoln (Eds.), *Handbook of qualitative research* (2nd ed.). Thousand Oaks, CA: Sage Publication.

Williams, B. (1978). *A sampler on sampling.* New York: Wiley.

Appendix A

Suggested Guide for Abstracting Research Studies

1. Complete bibliographic data: Include author, title, source, date, and pages.

2. Statement of the problem: Use direct quotes, if possible, to identify the area in which the study was conducted and purpose of the study.

3. Hypotheses: Use direct quotes to list hypotheses if they are presented.

4. Sample: Note how many subjects were in the actual sample, as well as characteristics (i.e., age level, socioeconomic status [SES], and geographic area). Note method of selecting or identifying sample).

5. Procedures: Outline actual steps taken in the study (i.e., sources of data, collection procedures).

6. Instruments: Note name(s) of instruments(s), reliability and validity of each. Summarize procedures used if new instrument was developed.

7. Time frame: Note time frame used in the study.

8. Method of analysis: Summarize statistical tests applied to the data or analytic method used.

9. Findings: Construct a concise statement of the most noteworthy findings.

10. Interpretations, conclusions   Note briefly the recommendations by the author-investigator regarding application of findings and future research.

11. General suggestions:

   1. Make notes regarding your own critique of each of the above parts, using contents of the present document.
   2. Avoid the need to return to the original source.
   3. Develop a hard copy or computerized filing system to speed retrieval.

Appendix B

Guide to Critique
of Philosophical Research

1. Is the topic to be explored, its breadth and scope, explicitly identified in the title of the dissertation? Or early in the introduction?
2. Are the purposes and aims of the inquiry clearly stated early in the introduction as well as in the methodology to be used?
3. Is the rationale justifying the inquiry convincing and regarded as worthwhile? Necessary? Useful? And not a duplication without new insights?
4. Does the organization of the inquiry build logically from one topic to the next?
5. Does the inquiry proceed through argumentation by interpretation rather than argumentation by empirical evidence as the major mode of discussion?
6. Is bibliographical data including the author's biases and perspective given if they are likely to influence the interpretation of the major themes developed in the argumentation? Is it necessary for this inquiry?
7. Are all major writings on the question or topic, pro and con, consulted in the presentation of possible views and/or approaches to its resolution? If not, is a rationale given for selection of certain authors over others?
8. Is there a consistency in the use of rhetoric and preservation of the selected author's views in context throughout the dissertation?
9. Are the strengths and weaknesses of opposing positions explicit in their exposition in the argumentation and resolution of the question?
10. Are assumptions and/or presuppositions identified underlying the major arguments or positions from which they were derived?
11. Do the arguments developed in the inquiry adhere to the assumptions of the positions from which they were derived?

12. Is it clear who the intended readers are to be addressed in the inquiry? Who is the audience for this polemic?
13. Is the proposal or answer derived through argumentation by interpretation convincing? And intelligible to the intended readers?
14. Are the aims and purposes of the dissertation accomplished?

Appendix C
Issues of Control and Validity: Quantitative Studies

CONTROL OF EXTRANEOUS VARIABLES BY DESIGN—AN EXAMPLE

An uncontrolled variable that greatly influences the results of a study is called an extraneous variable. Extraneous variables are those that lie outside the interest, or perhaps the control, of the researcher. There are usually a great number of these variables present, and they can often play an important role in affecting research results. (See the sample article at the end of this Appendix.)

Hoskins, C. N., Baker, S., Sherman, D., Bohlander, J., Bookbinder, M. Budin, W., Ekstrom, D., Kramer, C., & Maislin, G. (1996). Social support and patterns of adjustment to breast cancer. *Scholarly Inquiry for Nursing Practice: An International Journal, Vol. 10, No. 2* (pp. 99–122). New York: Springer Publishing Co.

A. Independent variables

   1. Marital support (symbolized by X_1)
   2. Functional status (symbolized by X_2)

      — vocational role
      — domestic role
      — social role

   3. Extramarital support (symbolized by X_3)

      — other adults
      — extended family

   4. Health care satisfaction (symbolized by X_4)

B.   Dependent variables (symbolized by Y_1, Y_2, Y_3, Y_4)

    1.   Emotional symptoms
    2.   Physical symptoms
    3.   Health status
    4.   Psychological well-being

C.   Controls of extraneous variables

The identified sources of extraneous variables were controlled primarily by five factors.

    1.   Research design

        —   longitudinal design to capture change over time
        —   research evidence to identify four phases of the breast cancer experience (i.e., diagnostic, post-surgery, adjuvant therapy, and ongoing recovery)
        —   data on current therapy and side effects were collected as these factors have a potential for contributing to variance in emotional and physical adjustment
        —   times of data collection were standardized

    2.   Variables

        —   clear conceptual definitions of the independent and dependent variables
        —   acceptable levels of validity and reliability from the present study sample
        —   instructions for completing the measures of the variables were standardized, thus maintaining little or no measurement error

    3.   Literature review

        —   an in-depth literature review with critique of studies, and citation of support for relationships between variables
        —   a clear theoretical framework, providing support for the hypotheses
        —   identification of variables, other than the independent variables, that could contribute to the variance in the dependent variables (i.e., functional status in vocational, domestic, and social roles that were hypothesized to contribute to the variance in emotional and physical adjustment)

    4.   Sample

        —   homogeneity in type of cancer (i.e., only subjects with early stage breast cancer were included in the study)
        —   subjects who had a history of cancer were excluded as responses to a recurrence vary from those to a first time diagnosis

— patients and partners who had a history of psychiatric hospitalization or drug abuse were excluded as emotional disability can contribute to the variance in such crises as a diagnosis of cancer

5. Data analyses

— missing data were maintained at a level below 10%, thus minimizing sample bias and measurement error
— a case management approach was used to maintain a relationship to subjects, thus maintaining low attrition
— appropriate statistical procedures were used for the level of data collected (i.e., nominal or continuous)

D. Extraneous variables not controlled

Not all extraneous variables can be controlled in human behavioral research. It is the responsibility, however, of the investigator to utilize the in-depth review of literature to identify as many extraneous variables as possible, then decide which ones have a sufficiently strong potential for contributing to the variance in the dependent variable(s) (i.e., emotional and physical adjustment). Such variables require control. Examples of extraneous variables that were not controlled are listed below. In a critique of the study by Northouse (1996), others are identified.

1. Research design

— the intervals between data collection times were not equal

2. Variables

— the type and length of surgery, reconstruction, and adjuvant therapy varied among patients

3. Sample

— the initial psychological status of the patients and partners was not measured
— the sample was drawn from the private practices of surgeons, leading to a homogeneous sample in terms of socioeconomic status, ethnicity, and heterosexual dyads

Northouse, L. L. (1996). Response to "social support and patterns of adjustment to breast cancer." *Scholarly Inquiry for Nursing Practice: An International Journal, 10*(2), 125–127.

The following is a critique of the article discussed in this Appendix by Laurel Northouse.

Social Support and Patterns of Adjustment to Breast Cancer

Carol Noll Hoskins, Ph.D., R.N., F.A.A.N.
Sonia Baker, Ph.D., R.N.
Deborah Sherman, Ph.D., R.N.
New York University

Jean Bohlander, Ph.D., R.N.
College Misericordia

Marilyn Bookbinder, Ph.D., R.N.
Memorial Sloan-Kettering Cancer Center

Wendy Budin, Ph.D., R.N.
Seton Hall University

David Ekstrom, Ph.D., R.N.
Pace University

Cynthia Knauer, M.S., R.N.
Beth Israel Medical Center-Petrie Division

Greg Maislin, M.S., M.A.
Biomedical Statistical Consulting,
Wynnewood, PA

The effect of marital support and support from other adults on the emotional and physical adjustment of 128 women with breast cancer was examined. Role function and satisfaction with health care also were evaluated as predictors of adjustment. Intact data series were obtained at 7-10 days, at 1, 2, 3, and 6 months, and 1 year postsurgery. Emotional adjustment could be predicted by satisfaction with a spouse's response to interactional and emotional needs and by support from other adults. The relationships were significant at concurrent times, across contiguous times, and predicting from the 7-10 day postsurgical period to both the 6-month and 1-year end points. Physical adjustment was not predicted by support but satisfaction with health care was predictive of perceived overall health status. Functional status in vocational, domestic, and social

Note. From "Social Support and Patterns of Adjustment to Breast Cancer," by C. N. Hoskins, S. Baker, D. Sherman, J. Bohlander, M. Bookbinder, W. Budin, D. Ekstrom, C. Knauer, and G. Maislin, 1996, *Scholarly Inquiry for Nursing Practice: An International Journal, 10*, pp. 99–123. Copyright 1996 by Springer Publishing Co. Reprinted with permission.

roles was significantly related to emotional and physical adjustment at all
phases with few exceptions.

Adjustment to breast cancer is reflected in behavioral responses that are emotional,
physical and cognitive. The need to study adjustment to breast cancer as a variable
response is strongly indicated in recent research (Ell, Nishimoto, Morvay, Mantell,
& Hamovitch, 1989; Iscoe, Williams, Szalai, & Osoba, 1991; Northouse, 1989a).
Some women treated for breast cancer report minimal negative responses (Krouse
& Krouse, 1982; Silberfarb, Maurer, & Crouthamel, 1980), or even positive effects
that promote support (Cohen, 1984; Wellisch, 1985). Others appear to be at risk in
terms of physical symptoms, role limitations, inadequate emotional support, and
difficulty with personal control that may last as long as 9-12 months postsurgery (Ell
et al., 1989).

The overall aim of the present study was to examine the central proposition that
inadequate support from the spouse and from other adults following surgery is
predictive of patients' self-reported (a) emotional adjustment, (b) physical adjustment, and (c) perceived health status over time. Alterations in ability to function in
the domestic, vocational, and social environments and degree of satisfaction with
health care were evaluated also as predictors of adjustment. The main propositions
are represented diagrammatically in one cross-section of the longitudinal design in
Figure 1.

PREDICTORS OF ADJUSTMENT

Since the 1970s, interest in social support has led to efforts to understand the nature
and meaning of the construct (Barrera, 1986; Dimond & Jones, 1983; Heitzmann
& Kaplan, 1988; House & Kahn, 1985; Norbeck, 1981; Rock, Green, Wise, & Rock,
1984; Stewart, 1989; Tilden, 1985). Although conceptualization and measurement
issues are debated in critical reviews, there is consensus that support plays an
important role in mitigating the negative psychosocial sequelae of an illness
(Bloom, 1982; Peters-Golden, 1982; Wortman, 1984; Wortman & Dunkel-Schetter,
1979). Schaefer, Coyne, and Lazarus (1981) note that persons who perceive
adequate support report fewer symptoms and less psychopathology in stressful
situations than those who perceive inadequate support. Well-being (Dunkel-
Schetter, 1984), lower levels of anxiety and depression, better social adjustment
(Dunkel-Schetter, 1984; Jamison, Wellisch, & Pasnau, 1978; Zemore & Shepel,
1989), and higher self-esteem (Feather & Wainstock, 1989) are outcomes of
adequate support.

The spouse often has been identified as the most pivotal person within the
patient's social support network; however, studies focusing on marital support are
limited (Jamison et al., 1978; Lichtman, 1982; Northouse, 1989b; Taylor, Lichtman,

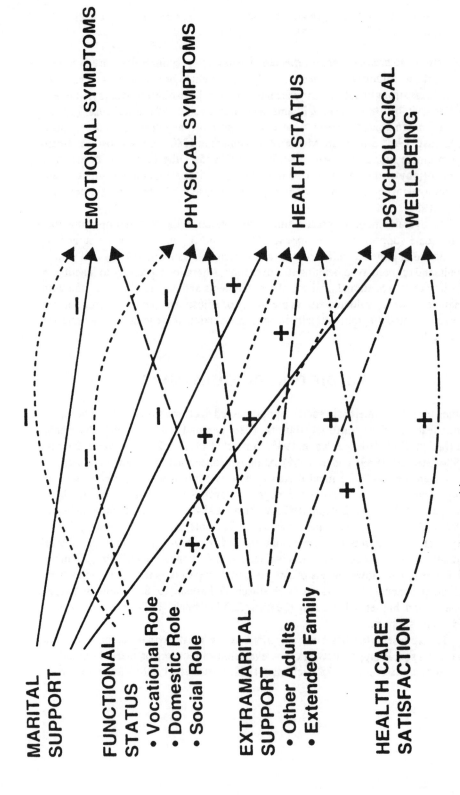

Figure 1. Diagram of main propositions

& Wood, 1985; Wellisch, 1985). The conceptualization and measurement of support in the marital relationship have varied from retrospective reports by 41 mastectomy patients who indicated that more understanding and support from a spouse were associated with better emotional adjustment (Jamison et al., 1978) to ratings of the spouse by 50 mastectomy patients on supportive behaviors (Northouse, 1988).

Social support and adjustment may influence each other (Jamison et al., 1978; Wortman & Dunkel-Schetter, 1979; Zemore & Shepel, 1989). Persons who are well adjusted to their illness often find it easier to elicit support (Bloom, 1982). As the most feared disease among healthy persons, cancer may lead, however, to stigmatization and avoidance behaviors. Peters-Golden (1982) noted from her interviews of 100 breast cancer patients and 100 disease-free individuals that 72% of the patients reported that they were treated differently after people knew they had cancer. They experienced less support than expected and cited it as the reason for difficulty in adjustment.

In addition to social support, potential predictors of adjustment include quality of relationship to the health care team, social integration (Loveys & Klaich, 1991), life stress unrelated to the cancer (Ell et al., 1989), time since diagnosis (Irvine, Brown, Crooks, Roberts, & Browne, 1991), and previous diagnosis of cancer.

The support network structure, including who provides support (Neuling & Winefield, 1988), context and type of support desired (Wellman, 1981), and length of time since diagnosis (Wortman & Dunkel-Schetter, 1979) all contribute to whether support is perceived as adequate. Although cancer patients may perceive information and advice from health care providers as supportive, the same input from family and friends may not be seen as helpful (Dunkel-Schetter, 1984)

Adjustment as an Ongoing Process

The impact of a diagnosis of cancer, effects of treatment, and uncertainty of cure tend to be chronic concerns, although some phases are characterized by more demands and stress than others. Jamison and associates (1978) noted that the period of maximum stress among 41 women who provided data in the pre- and post-mastectomy periods occurred between diagnosis and surgery. Northouse (1989b), in interviews of 50 mastectomy patients at 3 days, 30 days, and 18 months postsurgery, confirmed that the diagnostic and immediate postoperative periods are particularly stressful. Although Loveys and Klaich (1991) did not identify phase of illness in their semi-structured interviews of 79 women, the concerns identified most frequently were acceptance of the illness, treatment issues, social interaction or support, and changes in perspective on life, none of which is a time limited concern. The women, newly diagnosed with breast cancer within the previous 2½ years, indicated that the demands associated with the illness and treatment contributed to ongoing needs for information, decision making, and coping with physical changes, life change, uncertainty, and loss.

APPENDIX C

Adjustment to breast cancer has been measured by a number of emotional and physical responses: mental health (Ell et al., 1989), self-esteem, psychological symptoms, sexual dysfunction (Cella, 1987; Lasry, 1991), body image (Kemeny, Wellisch, & Schain, 1988; Krouse & Krouse, 1982), mood (Northouse, 1989a), psychosocial distress, and quality of life (Iscoe et al., 1991). Quality of life is considered to be an important indicator of adjustment and generally is associated with cognitive, social, physical, and emotional functioning (Shumaker, Anderson, & Czajkowski, 1990). It has been suggested, however, that conceptualization and measurement of quality of life should be broadened beyond functional status in these domains to include well-being and general health perception (Ware, 1990). The present study addresses this issue.

Other issues relevant to studies of women with breast cancer include limited internal validity due to lack of homogeneity in type of cancer, retrospective or a one-time measurement design, highly variable sample size, and absence of inclusion criteria. In the present study, the longitudinal design permitted the examination of two different types of hypotheses: (a) examination of the relations between predictors and outcomes of adjustment at each phase, considered separately, and (b) examination of the longitudinal dynamics of the relations over time.

Hypotheses

1. Patients who report less support in the marital relationship also report more problems with emotional and physical adjustment at the same and subsequent phase than do patients who report more support.

2. Patients who report more support from adults other than the spouse and from extended family report fewer problems with emotional and physical adjustment at the same and subsequent phase than do patients who report less support.

3. Patients reporting a higher degree of satisfaction with health care also report a perception of better overall health status at the same and subsequent phase.

4. Those patients who report difficulty in role function as a result of illness also report more problems with emotional and physical adjustment at the same and subsequent phase.

METHOD

Six assessments were scheduled at times that are consistent with events commonly associated with treatment and recovery for breast cancer (Baider & Kaplan De-Nour, 1984; Gotay, 1984; Northouse & Swain, 1987; Wilson & Morse, 1991): 7-10 days postsurgery, 1 month, 2 months, 3 months, 6 months, and 1 year postsurgery.

Sample

The sample was drawn from the practices of four breast surgeons at three major medical centers in the New York metropolitan area. Patients were accrued in the early phases of treatment. The criteria for inclusion in the study were no previous diagnosis of cancer, no history of psychiatric hospitalization or drug abuse, either married or living with a heterosexual partner, and able to read and understand English.

Data for 174 breast cancer patients were collected. Of these, 74% ($n = 128$) had sufficient data to be included in the analyses. When a score was missing for a respondent at a testing time but was present at the time before and the time after, the missing score was supplied by linear interpolation. Interpolated scores accounted for 2.6% of all scores available.

Detailed demographic and medical data were available for 120 of these 128 included subjects (94%) and for 21 of the 46 (46%) excluded subjects (Table 1). Among the included and excluded patients there were no significant differences in mean ages, lengths of present marriage, years of education, income, whether the patient was presently working, and family history of breast lesion.

Instruments

At each data collection point, the respondents completed four standardized inventories: the Partner Relationship Inventory [PRI] (Hoskins, 1988); the Psychosocial

TABLE 1. Demographic and Medical Characteristics

Demographic variables	Medical variables	
Caucasian	Surgical Procedure	
Mean Age	Breast Conserving Surgery	50.8%
51.0 years (SD = 9.9)	Non-breast Conserving Surgery	49.2%
	Reconstruction	52.0%
Mean Education	No Reconstruction	48.0%
14.8 years	Lymph Node Status	
	Positive lymph nodes	24.6%
Mean Length of Marriage	Negative lymph nodes	75.6%
25 years (SD = 11.5)	Data not available	N = 6
	Tumor Classification	
	< 2 cm	64.5%
	2–5 cm	23.4%
	> 5 cm	6.5%
	in situ	4.7%
	Adjuvant Therapy	
	Chemotherapy	47.0%
	Radiation therapy	49.0%
	Hormone treatment	41.0%

Adjustment to Illness Scale [PAIS] (Derogatis, 1983); the Profile of Adaptation to Life Clinical Scale [PAL-C] (Ellsworth, 1981); and the Self-Rated Health Subscale [SRHS] of the Multilevel Assessment Instrument [MAI] (Lawton, Moss, Fulcomer, & Kleban, 1982). The subscales of the measures and definitions are provided in Table 2.

The Partner Relationship Inventory was originally designed as a measure of need fulfillment and support in the marital relationship. Role theory provided the framework, which suggests that a mutually supportive relationship is based on congruency between partners in perceptions of one another's role in providing for needs to be met. When a major discrepancy occurs, whether it be in the perception of another's role, expectations of the other, or actual satisfaction of needs, the quality and supportive nature of the relationship are compromised.

The 40-item PRI has two subscales. The Emotional Needs subscale consists of 15 items and the Interactional Needs subscale, 25 items. The two subscales together comprise eight categories, each of which focuses on a specific domain of need. The PRI is self-administered, has a 4-point Likert response format, and requires the respondent to answer each item according to current feelings, thus tapping perceptions at a particular phase of illness. Two alternate forms of the PRI with equal levels of reliability were developed for repeated measurement in longitudinal designs.

Construct validity of the PRI was assessed originally by administering the short form of the Marital Adjustment Scale (Locke & Wallace, 1959) to the standardization sample of 52 couples, along with the initial 90-item long form of the PRI. The Pearson product-moment correlation coefficients between the Locke and Wallace marital adjustment score and scores for each of the PRI categories ranged between -.40 and -.75. Less satisfaction with need fulfillment, as reflected in higher scores, was related to lower levels of marital adjustment. A varimax rotated factor analysis supported a clear division of categories between two factors or subscales. Test-retest reliability when the inventory was administered on two occasions was supported by correlation coefficients between category scores that ranged between .84 and .95.

In the present study, the range in alpha coefficients across data collection times exceeded .90 for both Emotional Needs and Interactional Needs.

The Psychosocial Adjustment to Illness Scale is designed to measure seven domains of psychosocial adjustment (Derogatis, 1983). The PAIS consists of 46 items in a self-report format. Norms for the PAIS were developed for lung and breast cancer patients. Studies of discriminant validity among breast cancer patients yielded correlations between the total PAIS score of .81 for the Global Adjustment to Illness Scale, .60 for the SCL-90-R General Severity Index, and .69 for the Affect Balance Scale ($n = 27$). The reliability for the total PAIS score was .86.

The alpha coefficients across data collection times for the seven domains in the present study were .42 to .73 for Extended Family Relationships, .62 to .71 for Health Care Orientation, .64 to .75 for Vocational Environment, .66 to .77 for Domestic Environment, .83 to .85 for Social Environment, and .86 to .89 for

TABLE 2. Definitions and Measures of Variables

Variables	Definitions	Subscales
Predictors		
Marital support	Need for affection, emotional security and stability in the relationship; appreciation by the partner.	Emotional needs
	Need for open communication of feelings and perceptions; congruency in thinking; shared interests and companionship.	Interaction needs
Extramarital support	Closeness to adults other than the spouse.	Close interpersonal relationships
	Communication; interest in interacting; physical and social dependency.	Extended family relations
Health care satisfaction	Satisfaction with information about the illness and interaction with health-care providers; attitude toward personal care.	Health care orientation
Functional status	Impact of illness on job performance, interest, and satisfaction; lost time and other impairments.	Vocational environment
	Financial aspects of the illness; quality of relationships and communication; impact of physical impairments.	Domestic environment
	Effect of illness on leisure interests and activities in the 'individual', 'family', and 'social' settings	Social environment
Outcomes		
Emotional adjustment	Feelings of uneasiness or tension.	Negative emotions
	Feelings of being involved, useful, and of self-esteem.	Psychological well-being
	Dysphoric thoughts and feelings as a result of the illness and its sequelae.	Psychological distress
Physical adjustment	Frequency and intensity of physical symptoms	Physical symptoms
Health status	Expected health status at a given phase.	Better health
	Absence of physical problems.	No problems

Psychological Distress (Murphy, 1994). The low reliability of .42 for Extended Family Relationships may be due to the diversity of focus in the items, i.e., contact, interest in being together, availability for dependency needs, and general quality of the relationship.

The Profile of Adaptation to Life Clinical Scale also measures domains of psychological adjustment and physical outcomes. The scale is a 41-item self-report inventory sensitive to variations over time and to counseling intervention. The initial scale (PAL-R) consisted of 154 items to reflect a wide range of adjustment and functioning (Ellsworth, 1979b). It was administered initially and 3 months later to groups receiving various treatments or training in such modalities as conscious control of internal states through guided imagery ($n = 1,738$). The items retained in the clinical form of the scale (PAL-C) were selected according to the criteria of sensitivity to pre- and post-treatment change, ability to distinguish between groups known to differ in adjustment (discriminant validity), and salience of the item for measuring an adjustment domain based on factor analyses. A series of factor analyses performed on the groups separately identified the dimensions of adjustment common to all groups (Ellsworth, 1979). In studies of discriminant validity, the subscales of Negative Emotions, Psychological Well-Being, and Physical Symptoms were the best discriminators between groups. Criterion-related validity was established by significant correlations between self and other ratings, ranging between .20 and .86. Test-retest reliabilities were .80 and above.

In the present study, the alpha coefficient at all data collection points exceeded .90 for Close Interpersonal Relationships and for Negative Emotions; .75 for Psychological Well-Being; and .83 for Physical Symptoms.

The Multilevel Assessment Instrument was designed originally to measure well-being among older persons using domains of physical health, activities of daily living, cognition, time use, social interaction, personal adjustment, and perceived environment. The Self-Report Health Scale, one of three subscales within the domain of physical health, consists of four items to assess overall health status.

Validity and reliability estimates were derived from data collected from samples of older adults ($N = 590$). Summary ratings for each of the seven domains were obtained by consensus between an interviewer and a clinician. Validity was supported by a correlation of .67 between the summary domain for physical health and the health scale, and by a correlation of .63 between the ratings by the interviewer and clinician. Reliability of the health scale was supported by an internal consistency coefficient of .76 and test-retest of .92 at 3 weeks.

Factor analytic evaluation of the health scale in the present study yielded two factors, each consisting of two items (Merrifield & Hoskins, 1993). Reliability estimates from inter-item correlation coefficients for perceived health status with Factor I (Better Health) were .60, and with Factor II (No Problems), .69. Conceptually consistent with the notion of perceived health status in the present study, the health scale also could be administered on repeated occasions.

The means and standard deviations for the subscales as used in the present study are presented in Table 3.

TABLE 3. Possible Range for Subscale Scores, and Actual Ranges in Means and Standard Deviations Across Six Data Collection Times

Subscale	Possible Range	M	SD
Interactional needs	25–100	41.04–52.71	6.33–16.68
Emotional needs	15.60	23.92–27.27	5.82–9.97
Close interpersonal relationships*	5–20	16.39–17.06	3.26–3.92
Extended family relations	1–20	5.98–6.16	1.41–1.98
Health care orientation	1–32	12.77–13.46	3.03–3.45
Vocational environment	1–24	8.13–11.69	2.42–3.28
Domestic environment	1–32	10.96–12.88	3.04–3.36
Social environment	1–24	8.10–12.59	3.21–4.37
Negative emotions	5–20	13.01–14.26	4.06–4.21
Psychological distress	1–28	11.51–13.16	3.12–3.60
Psychological well-being*	5–20	15.76–17.07	3.26–4.11
Physical symptoms	7–28	11.69–12.65	1.10–1.24
Better health*	2–6	4.14–5.92	1.09–1.25
No health problems*	2–7		

*Scored in positive direction, i.e., a higher score indicates a more positive adjustment. A higher score on the other subscales indicates a lower level of adjustment or more problems.

Procedure

Approval for the study was obtained from the institutional review boards of three medical centers. Surgeons who agreed to refer patients to the study screened the patient either at the time of the first office visit or postsurgery. The medical records for patients who met the criteria and were referred to the study were reviewed by the office staff to determine previous history of cancer, psychiatric hospitalization, and English ability. The initial contact by an investigator with a patient who met the criteria occurred either in the surgeon's office or hospital setting. If the patient was interested in participating, the consent form was explained and signed. The four inventories, instructions for completion of the inventories, and a demographic data sheet were given to the patient. The baseline medical data were obtained from the medical record; ongoing information was obtained from the record and the patient.

A case management approach was used in the interest of maintaining rapport and sensitivity to the subject, familiarity with the patient's status, and minimal attrition. The investigator who made the initial contact with the patient followed her throughout the 1-year period of data collection. The four project investigators, each responsible for a caseload of patients, consisted of the principal investigator, two doctoral students in nursing, and a clinical nurse specialist in oncology. The investigators mailed the inventories with a personalized letter at each data collection time. Form letters1 appropriate to each time period had been developed by the principal investigator. Each set of inventories was accompanied by standardized instructions and a stamped envelope for return to the project office. The investigators also collected information on current therapy and side effects for each data collection time from the patient and medical record.

Data Analysis

Two of the four standardized inventories completed by respondents at each data collection point, the PAIS and the PRI, contained items differing in directionality and were reverse-scored. The constituent subscales of the four inventories were scored for each respondent at each point. Plots of the distributions of the variables at each point in time revealed departures from normality for some subscales. In most cases, these differences were significant, with $p < .0001$, using Shapiro-Wilk statistics.

There were no apparent patterns of association between testing time and means, standard deviations or skewness. Thus, scores on all predictor and outcome scales were normalized prior to parametric statistical analyses (Blom, 1958). Normal scores were computed as follows: The data were ranked, then the rank scores were used in the order statistics for the normal distribution (Tukey, 1962). T-scores were computed by multiplying the normal score by 10 and adding 50, so that the grand means and standard deviations were 50 and 10, respectively.

Tests of the hypotheses proceeded in four steps. First, the four hypotheses were tested for contemporaneous ("zero time lag") relationships between predictor and outcome variables at each phase. Pearson correlation coefficients were computed between the predictor set and the outcome set at each of six data collection points, i.e., 7-10 days to 1 year postsurgery. In order to protect against capitalization on chance (arising from the large number of coefficients evaluated at each point), Bonferroni significance tests were utilized for each of the correlation matrices. To reach a Bonferroni significance level of $p < .05$ (.01), the nominal p-value had to be smaller than .05 divided by the number of unique correlations being simultaneously tested.

Second, the hypotheses were tested for first-order lagged effects between predictor and outcome variables. Lagged relationships were evaluated by means of a series of canonical analyses (Cohen & Cohen, 1983), which drew on the entire predictor set at each point and on the entire outcome set at the immediately subsequent point. In each canonical procedure, a principal components analysis was performed for the predictor and outcome sets, yielding one or more pairs of canonical variates. Overall significance of the predictor/outcome relationship was evaluated by Wilks' lambda and its associated F-test. For each significant pair of canonical variates, the principal canonical loadings for both predictors and outcome variables were calculated. The global effect size was indexed by the canonical correlation coefficient, and all significant univariate tests were compiled for variables in the outcome set.

Third, to gauge the status of the hypotheses across the duration of the entire study period, each hypothesis was evaluated in a final canonical analysis that drew predictor variables from the 7-10-day point and outcome variables from both 6 months and 1 year postsurgery.

RESULTS

For each data collection point, contemporaneous relationships between Emotional and Physical Adjustment and Marital Support from the first hypothesis are given in Table 4. Correlations between variables operationalizing Emotional Adjustment and those indexing Marital Support are moderately large, reaching statistical significance at most points. Further, the signs of all *r* values for these relationships are as predicted. There is no significant relationship between Physical Adjustment and Marital Support.

Tests of the contemporaneous relationships as predicted by Hypothesis 2 indicate Emotional Adjustment (indexed by Negative Emotions) is inversely related to Support from Other Adults (Close Interpersonal Relationships), reaching significance at all phases (see Table 5). Emotional Adjustment (indexed by Psychological Well-Being) is directly related also to support from Close Interpersonal Relations, significantly so at all points. For both these sets of variables, the effect sizes are moderately large and the signs of all *r* values at all points are as predicted. Emotional Adjustment (Psychological Well-Being and Negative Emotions) is correlated with support from Extended Family Relations at specifc phases. As in the tests of Hypothesis 1, the Physical Adjustment outcome is not predicted by any predictors at any point, with the exception of 2 months.

In the tests of Hypothesis 3, the two measures of Overall Health Status (Better Health and No Problems) are correlated significantly with Satisfaction with Health Care (Health Care Orientation) at all phases, with the exception of 1 month and 1 year for the Better Health outcome and at the 7-10-day phase for No Problems (see Table 6). Taking into account the directionality of each scale and the sign of the Pearson coefficient, this indicates that less salutary attitudes toward the health care system and toward personal care are likely to indicate more health-related problems.

Tests of contemporaneous relationships predicted in Hypothesis 4 also yielded statistically significant results for most criteria and at most phases (see Table 7). The correlations are moderately large and the signs of all *r* values are as predicted. The predictors are significantly correlated with the physical adjustment outcome at all phases, with the exception of Vocational Environment at 7-10 days and 1 month and Social Environment at 1 year.

In the second step of data analysis, the five lagged canonical analyses (see Table 8) all yielded statistically significant results. Generally, from one point to the next, the canonical R^2 values for the first canonical variates ranged from 52%-61%. Thus, a substantial proportion of variance in the adjustment outcome set was accounted for by its linear association with the single canonical variate from the predictor set.

For the first canonical variate analyses, the eight predictor variables (comprising the support and role function domains) strongly load onto a canonical variate that predicts the three aspects of Emotional Adjustment and at least two aspects of Physical Adjustment in all five analyses. The three outcome variables comprising Emotional Adjustment strongly load onto a first canonical variate in all five analyses.

TABLE 4. Tests of Hypothesis 1: Correlations Between Emotional and Physical Adjustment and Marital Support Among Patients Treated for Breast Cancer

Variable Pairs	Data Collection Points					
	7–10 days (N = 127)	1- month (N = 128)	2- month (N = 128)	3- month (N = 128)	6-month (N = 128)	1-year (N = 121)[a]
I. Emotional Adjustment (Negative emotions)						
Marital Support						
{Emotional needs)	.24	.23*	.40**	.28*	.47**	.50**
{Interaction needs)	.22	.14	.47**	.25	.44**	.35**
II. Emotional Adjustment (Psychological well-being)						
Marital Support						
{Emotional needs)	−.32**	−.16	−.35**	−.32**	−.37**	−.35**
{Interaction needs)	−.39**	−.22	−.41**	−.34**	−.36**	−.29*
III. Physical Adjustment (Physical symptoms)						
Marital Support						
{Emotional needs)	.13	−.04	.23	.06	.20	.20
{Interaction needs)	.14	.11	.26	.08	.17	.20

Bonferroni tests: *p < .05. **p < .01.
[a]Sample size equal to N = 127 at 7–10 days and N = 121 at one year since interpolation using adjacent values not possible.

TABLE 5. Tests of Hypothesis 2: Correlations Between Emotional and Physical Adjustment and Extramarital Support Among Patients Treated for Breast Cancer

			Data Collection Points			
Variable Pairs	7-10 days ($N = 128$)	1-month ($N = 128$)	2-month ($N = 128$)	3-month ($N = 128$)	6-month ($N = 128$)	1-year ($N = 121$)[a]
I. Emotional Adjustment (Negative emotions) Extramarital Support						
(Close interpersonal relations)	-.29*	-.24*	-.43**	-.39**	-.46**	-.51**
(Extended family relations)	.20	.21	.28*	.25	.22	.21
II. Emotional Adjustment (Psychological well-being) Extramarital Support						
(Close interpersonal relations)	.43**	.39**	.56**	.53**	.49**	.55**
(Extended family relations)	-.28*	-.19	-.28*	-.27	-.16	-.44**
III. Physical Adjustment (Physical symptoms) Extramarital Support						
(Close interpersonal relations)	-.20	-.15	-.15	-.03	.15	-.23
(Extended family relations)	.09	.14	.30*	.13	.25	.12

Bonferroni tests: *$p < .05$.   **$p < .01$.
[a]Sample size equal to $N = 121$ at one year since interpolation using adjacent values not possible.

TABLE 6. Tests of Hypothesis 3: Correlations Between Overall Health Status and Health Care Satisfaction Among Patients Treated for Breast Cancer

			Data collection points			
Variable pairs	7-10 days ($N = 128$)	1-month ($N = 128$)	2-month ($N = 128$)	3-month ($N = 128$)	6-month ($N = 128$)	1-year ($N = 121$)[a]
I. Overall Health Status						
(Better health)	-.27*	-.23	-.30**	-.39**	-.30**	-.23
(No problems)	-.25	-.26*	-.38**	-.34**	-.37**	-.36**
Health Care Satisfaction						
(Health care orientation)						

Bonferroni tests: *$p < .05$.   **$p < .01$.

[a] Sample size equal to $N = 121$ at one year since interpolation using adjacent values not possible.

TABLE 7. Tests of Hypothesis 4: Correlations Between Emotional and Physical Adjustment and Role Function Among Patients Treated for Breast Cancer

	Data collection points					
Variable pairs	7-10 days (N = 127)	1-month (N = 128)	2-month (N = 128)	3-month (N = 127)	6-month (N = 127)	1-year (N = 121)[a]
I. Emotional Adjustment (Negative emotions) Role Function						
(Vocational environment)	.19	.24	.28	.33*	.37**	.28
(Domestic environment)	.26	.35**	.46**	.46**	.51**	.47**
(Social environment)	.28	.32*	.33**	.38**	.38**	.33*
II. Emotional Adjustment (Psychological well-being) Role Function						
(Vocational environment)	-.18	-.37**	-.44**	-.54**	-.53**	-.30
(Domestic environment)	-.22	-.32*	-.48**	-.48**	-.48**	-.39**
(Social environment)	.29*	-.43**	-.51**	-.47**	-.41**	-.42**
III. Emotional Adjustment (Psychological distress) Role Function						
(Vocational environment)	.29	.25	.43**	.48**	.52**	.44**
(Domestic environment)	.29*	.45**	.54**	.60**	.58**	.53**
(Social environment)	.36**	.42**	.47**	.57**	.52**	.40**
IV. Physical Adjustment (Physical symptoms) Role Function						
(Vocational environment)	.20	.26	.35**	.42**	.43**	.39**
(Domestic environment)	.36**	.36**	.43**	.42**	.46**	.34**
(Social environment)	.33**	.39**	.41**	.37**	.45**	.28

Bonferroni tests: *$p < .05$. **$p < .01$.
[a]Sample size equal to $N = 127$ at 7-10 days and $N = 121$ at one year since interpolation using adjacent values not possible; $N = 127$ at 3 months and 6 months due to an additional missing value.

TABLE 8. Sumary of Significant Findings From Canonical Analyses Lagged Across Contiguous DataCollection Points. Eight Predictors From the Antecedent Point Are Entered With Six Outcome Variables From the Subsequent Point ($N = 123$)

Lag Time	Predictor	CV	Outcome	CV
7–10 days–1 mo $R^2 = .55$ $p = <.0001$	Vocational environment Domestic environment Social environment Close relationships Extended family Emotional needs Interaction needs Health care	.69[a] .70 .76 −.42 .74 .45 .43 .45	Negative emotions Psych distress Psych well-being No problems Physical symptoms	.46 .60 −.77 −.66 .35
1 mo–2 mos $R^2 = .52$ $p = < .0001$	Vocational environment Domestic environment Social environment Close relationships Extended family Health care	.55 .72 .79 −.44 .41 .70	Negative emotions Psych distress Psych well-being No problems Physical symptoms	.64 .82 −.74 −.77 .59
2 mos–3 mos $R^2 = .60$ $p = < .0001$	Vocational environment Domestic environment Social environment Close relationships Extended family Health care Emotional needs Interaction needs	.71 .82 .75 −.48 .46 .62 .46 .51	Negative emotions Psych distress Psych well-being No problems Better health	.65 .78 −.84 −.65 −.42
3 mos–6 mos $R^2 = .61$ $p = < .0001$	Vocational environment Domestic environment Social environment Close relationships Extended family Health care Emotional needs Interaction needs	.85 .83 .86 −.48 .42 .60 .32 .35	Negative emotions Psych distress Psych well-being No problems Physical symptoms	.53 .70 −.78 −.73 .54
6 mos–1 yr $R^2 = .56$ $p = < .0001$	Vocational environment Domestic environment Social environment Close relationships Extended family Health care Emotional needs Interaction needs	.68 .81 .57 −.69 .35 .62 .80 .75	Negative emotions Psych distress Psych well-being No problems Physical symptoms	.79 .85 −.72 −.57 .57

[a]Structure Coefficients, i.e., correlations between the first canonical variate and the original variables. Coefficients of .30 or higher are reported as meaningful (Pedhazur, 1991. p. 732).

The canonical analyses lagged across contiguous time points support the proposition that women who report more support, i.e., from the marital relationship, from adults other than the spouse, and from the health care system, report fewer problems with emotional and physical adjustment at each subsequent phase than do patients who report less support. Also, women who are better able to carry out their roles within the Vocational, Domestic, and Social Environments tend to report less psychological distress, a greater sense of well-being, and fewer health problems at the subsequent phase.

A second canonical variate was statistically significant ($p = .04$) for the 7-10-day to 1 month lagged analysis. This variate shared an additional 15% of variance with the adjustment outcome variate. Predictor variables with structure coefficients greater than .30 for this second variate included Domestic Environment (.34), Social Environment (.34), and Health Care (.44). Outcome variables with structure coefficients greater than .30 included Physical Symptoms (.84), Better Health (-.67), Psychological Distress (.44), and Negative Emotions (.40). Thus, the second canonical variate placed greater emphasis on physical outcomes compared to the first canonical variate.

In general, second canonical variates were statistically significant for the remaining four lagged analyses ($p < .02$). The additional shared variance was 23%, 28%, 28%, and 28% for 1 to 2 months, 2 to 3 months, 3 to 4 months, and 6 months to 1 year, respectively. Only for the 2 to 3 months analyses was a third canonical variate statistically significant ($p = .05$).

In the third step of data analysis, predictions for Hypotheses 1 and 2 were tested across the 7-10-days to 6 months period and across the 7-10-days to 1 year period. Results are given in Figures 2-5. Figure 2 shows that, as implied in Hypothesis 1, an underlying canonical variate (Marital Support) correlates strongly with both Emotional Needs and Interaction needs at 7-10 days. Similarly, a second canonical variate (Emotional Adjustment) is correlated strongly with both Negative Emotions and Psychological Well-Being at 6 months. The structure coefficients between variables and their canonical variates at 1 year are similar to those found at 6 months (see Figure 3).

The canonical correlation between Emotional Adjustment at 6 months post-surgery and Marital Support at 7-10 days is .436, i.e., 19% of the variance is shared by a linear combination of the two predictors, a moderate effect size that holds over a 6-month time lag. In Figure 3, it may be seen that adjustment at 1 year also is predicted by Marital Support at 7-10 days. The canonical correlation is .531; 28% of the variation in the variates created from Emotional and Physical Adjustment at 1 year and Marital Support at 7-10 days was shared.

The second main hypothesis predicted a relationship between adjustment and support from adults other than the spouse. Support from Close Interpersonal Relationships and Extended Family at 7-10 days load strongly onto the first canonical variate (see Figure 4). Further, the two variables indexing Emotional Adjustment at 6 months (Negative Emotions and Psychological Well-Being) load

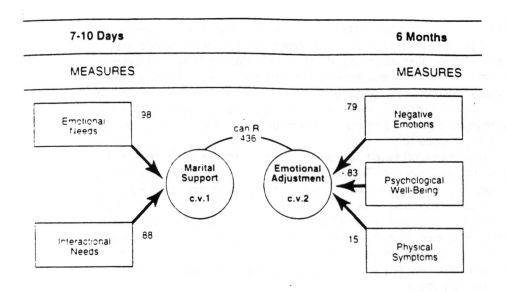

Wilks Lambda = .80; F = 4.89; (6,242); p = < 0.0001

Figure 2. Marital support at one-week post-surgery predicts emotional adjustment at six-month outcome in 126 patients with breast cancer

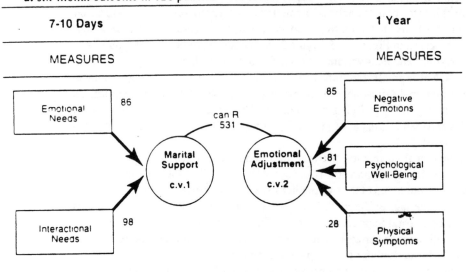

Wilks Lambda = .71; F = 6.92; (6,226); p = < 0.0001

Figure 3. Marital support at one-week post-surgery predicts emotional adjustment at one-year outcome in 118 patients with breast cancer

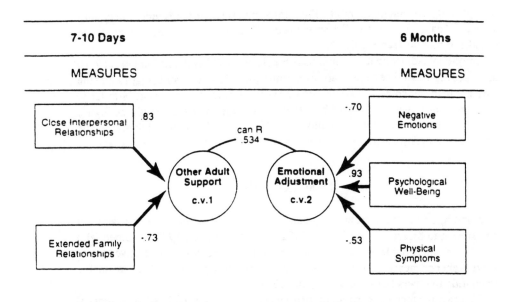

Wilks' Lambda = .69; $F = 8.37$; (6,246); $p = < 0.0001$

Figure 4. Support from other adults at one-week post-surgery predicts emotional adjustment at six-month outcome in 128 patients with breast cancer

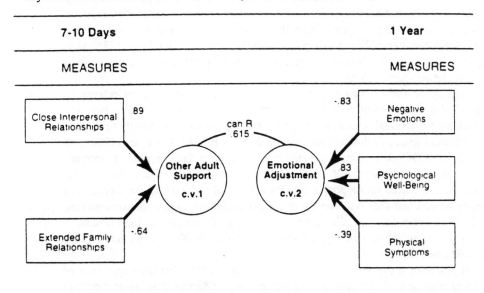

Wilks' Lambda = .60; $F = 10.96$; (6,230); $p = < 0.0001$

Figure 5. Support from other adults at one-week post-surgery predicts emotional adjustment at one-year outcome in 120 patients with breast cancer

strongly onto the canonical variate. Physical Symptoms also loads moderately onto the second canonical variate. The structure coefficients at 1 year are similar to those found at 6 months (see Figure 5).

Emotional Adjustment at 6 months is predicted by Other Adult Support at 7-10 days (see Figure 4). The canonical correlation equals .534, indicating that 29% of the variance in the outcome set variate is shared with the predictor set variate. Similarly, adjustment at 1 year is predicted by Other Adult Support at 7-10 days (see Figure 5). The overall canonical correlation is .615; i.e., 38% of the variance in the Emotional Adjustment variate is shared with the Other Adult Support variate.

DISCUSSION

The findings from the present study confirm that social support is a key factor in adjustment to breast cancer (Bloom, 1982; Dunkel-Schetter, 1984). Women who are able to talk about feelings and concerns with a spouse, friend or relative tend to score higher on measures of adjustment than patients who report that they are unable to confide in others (Zemore & Shepel, 1989).

Contrary to other work, marital support was clearly conceptualized in the present study as the perceived degree of satisfaction with a spouse's response to emotional and interactional needs during the diagnostic, postsurgical, adjuvant therapy, and ongoing recovery phases of breast cancer. Flexibility in responding to changing events is required from an adjustment point of view and can be captured only by means of a longitudinal design. Difficulty between partners in redefining expectations of one another during illness and treatment has clear implications for emotional well-being. Few investigators (Silberfarb et al., 1980; Vess, 1986) have addressed the need for flexibility in role expectations as the functional level within the ill partner changes over time.

Among the women in the present study, the need for emotional support from the spouse did not lessen over time. In fact, the strength of the relationship between inadequate emotional support and negative emotions escalated steadily between 1 month and 1 year, a finding consistent with those of Ell and colleagues (1989) and Northouse (1989a). Similarly, dissatisfaction with a partner's response to interactional needs was predictive of Negative Emotions and Psychological Well-Being. The enormous need for support in both the emotional and interactional domains in relation to the demands associated with diagnosis of breast cancer, decision making related to treatment, side effects, and uncertainty of cure are not time limited, a finding consistent with findings of Baider and Kaplan De-Nour (1984) and Loveys and Klaich (1991).

It has been suggested (Cohen, 1984; Wellisch, 1985) that the experience of cancer may actually provide a stimulus for more effective communication and attention to support. The findings from the present study indicate, however, that those women who report dissatisfaction with emotional need fulfillment initially continue to perceive inadequate support and to experience adjustment problems, supporting the findings that initial psychological status is predictive of subsequent emotional adjustment to breast cancer (Ell et al., 1988; Iscoe et al., 1991). Implications include the importance of identifying women at risk through the use of valid and reliable measures such as the constituent subscales of the Marital Support variate.

The need for support outside the marital relationship also increased over time, a finding consistent with that of other investigators who have noted that cancer is a chronic disease (Lewis, 1990; Schaefer et al., 1981) with ongoing demands (Varrichio, 1990). Again, the importance of valid and reliable assessments of extramarital support across time is reinforced.

Consistent with this notion, satisfaction with information and support from physicians and nurses enhances a more positive perception of global health status. Support by health care professionals is basic to trust and confidence in the treatment process (Loveys & Klaich, 1991) and must be maintained in the interest of promoting positive adjustment.

Functional status within the settings of job, home, and social environment were inversely related to both emotional and physical adjustment, a finding consistent with those of other investigators (Silberfarb et al., 1980; Vess, 1986). These relationships may operate in a reciprocal manner, i.e., physical symptoms contribute to impairment. Women need to be counseled to request treatment times and to monitor side effects in the interest of limiting dysfunction and creating a sense of empowerment. As integral parts of a family unit, many women were preoccupied with the impact of their diagnosis and treatment on both their spouse and children. A family systems perspective (Lewis, Hammond, & Woods, 1993; Rait & Lederberg, 1990) is extremely useful when counseling a woman to request and accept help from her family when needed and to enhance her understanding of the experience of other family members.

Implications for nursing practice include :

- To provide information relevant to the options for treatment at key points in time. Collaboration with health care providers in making informed decisions must be a part of the treatment process.

- To conduct assessments that are comprehensive, including resources for support and level of functioning in all facets of the patient's life.

- To acknowledge differences among the patient, her family, other support networks, and health care professionals. Decision-making needs to be based on recognition of differences in both immediate and long-range objectives.

- To plan educational and supportive interventions that are responsive to needs as they vary over time in the interest of promoting long-term adjustment.

- To identify and treat women who are at risk in terms of satisfactory adjustment to breast cancer. Implement useful, cost-effective interventions to these women that address both educational and support needs at key phases of treatment.

• To recognize that many women may not have traditional support networks and, therefore, may need strengthening of other sources of support.

• To educate all women in both self-care and preventive methods, such as breast self-examination.

The profound psychosocial impact of breast cancer affects both the woman and her family, often extending beyond the course of active medical treatment. In the present longitudinal study, women with breast cancer and their spouses were followed for 1 year. Four phases of emotional and physical adjustment were identifed for patients; diagnostic, postsurgical, adjuvant therapy, and ongoing recovery. Predictors of emotional and physical adjustment were determined for each group. It was found that women with breast cancer and their spouses experience similar and yet different distress along the diagnostic, treatment, and recovery trajectory (Hoskins et al., 1996). Findings indicated the enormous importance of education, effective communication, support, and other interventions in the interest of promoting mental health in both the woman and her spouse over time.

Further research would use the rich data base to design and produce eight sets of psychoeducational materials, one set of four for women and a second set of four for partners. Little is known about which kinds or combinations of interventions are most effective in promoting adjustment. The efficacy of structured psychoeducation has not been examined, nor has the impact of phase-specific content on emotional and physical adjustment been studied in a systematic clinical trial. Further research would fill the gap in our knowledge of which modes of psychosocial interventions are most effective and for which categories of patients and families.

REFERENCES

Baider, L., & Kaplan De-Nour, A.K. (1984). Couples' reactions and adjustment to mastectomy. *International Journal of Psychiatry and Medicine, 14,* 265-276.

Barrera, M. (1986). Distinctions between social support concepts, measures, and models. *American Journal of Community Psychology, 14,* 413-445.

Blom, G. (1958). *Statistical estimates and transformed beta variables.* New York: Wiley.

Bloom, J. (1982). Social support, accommodation to stress, and adjustment to breast cancer. *Social Science & Medicine, 16,* 1329-1338.

Cella, D. (1987). Cancer survival: Psychosocial and public issues. *Cancer Investigations, 5,* 59-67.

Cohen, J., & Cohen, P. (1983). *Applied multiple regression/correlation analysis for the behavioral sciences.* (2nd ed.). Hillsdale, NJ: Lawrence Erlbaum.

Cohen, R.S. (1984). *The impact of the diagnosis and treatment of breast cancer on the close relationship process.* (Unpublished doctoral dissertation, UCLA, Los Angeles).

Derogatis, L.R. (1983). *The psychosocial adjustment to illness scale.* Baltimore, MD: Clinical Psychometric Research.

Dimond, M., & Jones, S. (1983). Social support: A review and theoretical integration. In P. Chinn (Ed.), *Advances in nursing theory development* (pp. 235-249). Rockville, MD: Aspen.

Dunkel-Schetter, C. (1984). Social support and cancer: Findings based on patient interviews and their implications. *Journal of Social Issues, 40,* 77-79.

Ell. K., Nishimoto, R., Morvay, T., Mantell, J., & Hamovitch, M. (1989). A longitudinal analysis of psychological adaptation among survivors of cancer. *Cancer, 63,* 406-413.

Ellsworth, R. B. (1979). *The PARS Scale: A measure of Personal Adjustment and Role Skills.* Roanoke, VA: Institute for Program Evaluation.

Ellsworth, R. B. (1981). *Profile of adaptation to life clinical scale.* Palo Alto, CA: Consulting Psychologists.

Feather, B.L., & Wainstock, J.M. (1989). Perception of postmastectomy patients. Part 1. The relationships between social support and network providers. *Cancer Nursing, 2,* 293-300.

Gotay, C.C. (1984). The experience of cancer during early and advanced stages: The views of patients and their mates. *Social Science and Medicine, 18,* 605-613.

Heitzman, C., & Kaplan, R. (1988). Assessment of methods for measuring social support. *Health Psychology, 7,* 75-109.

Hoskins, C.N. (1988). *The partner relationship inventory.* Palo Alto, CA: Consulting Psychologists.

Hoskins, C.N., Baker, S., Bookbinder, M., Budin, W., Ekstrom, D., Knauer, C., Maislin, G., Sherman, D., & Steelman-Bohlander, J. (1996). Adjustment among spouses of women with breast cancer. *Journal of Psychosocial Oncology, 14*(1), 41-69.

House, J., & Kahn, R. (1985). Measures and concepts of social support. In S. Cohen & S. Syme (Eds.), *Social support and health.* (pp. 83-108). New York: Academic Press.

Irvine, D., Brown, B., Crooks, D., Roberts, J., & Browne, G. (1991). Psychosocial adjustment in women with breast cancer. *Cancer,* 1097-1117.

Iscoe, N.J., Williams, J.P., Szalai, J.P., & Osoba, D. (1991). Prediction of psychosocial distress in patients with cancer. In D. Osoba (Ed.), *Effect of cancer on quality of life* (pp. 41-59). Boston: CRC Press.

Jamison, K.R., Wellisch, D.K., & Pasnau, R.O. (1978). Psychosocial aspects of mastectomy. I. The women's perspective. *American Journal of Psychiatry, 136,* 432-436.

Kemeny, M.M., Wellisch, D.K., & Schain, W.S. (1988). Psychosocial outcomes in a randomized surgical trial for treatment of primary breast cancer. *Cancer, 62,* 1231-1237.

Krouse, H., & Krouse, J. (1982). Cancer as crisis: The critical elements of adjustment. *Nursing Research, 31,* 96-101.

Lasry, J. (1991). Women's sexuality following breast cancer. In D. Osoba (Ed.), *Effect of cancer on quality of life* (pp. 215-227). Boston: CRC Press.

Lawton, M.P., Moss, M.S., Fulcomer, M., & Kleban, M.H. (1982). A research and service oriented multilevel assessment instrument. *Journal of Gerontology, 37,* 91-99.

Lewis, F.M. (1990). Strengthening family supports. *Cancer, 65,* 752-759.

Lewis, F.M., Hammond, M.A., & Woods, N.F. (1993). The family's functioning with chronic illness in the mother: The spouse's perspective. *Social Science and Medicine, 29,* 1261-1269.

Lichtman, R.G. (1982). *Close relationships after breast cancer.* (Unpublished doctoral dissertation, UCLA, Los Angeles).

Locke, H., & Wallace, K. (1959). Short marital adjustment and prediction tests: Their reliability and validity. *Marriage and Family Living, 21,* 251-255.

Loveys, B.J., & Klaich, K. (1991). Breast cancer: Demands of illness. *Oncology Nursing Forum, 18,* 75-79.

Merrifield, P., & Hoskins, C.N. (1993). Factor analyses and reliability estimates for the self-rated health scale. (Unpublished data)

Murphy, G. (1994). *Psychosocial adjustment to illness: An examination of measures.* (Unpublished doctoral dissertation, New York University, NY)

Neuling, S.J., & Winefield, H.R. (1988). Social support and recovery after surgery for breast cancer: Frequency and correlates of supportive behaviors by family, friends and surgeon. *Social Science and Medicine, 27,* 385-392.

EXEMPLAR RESPONSE

Response to "Social Support and Patterns of Adjustment to Breast Cancer"

Laurel L. Northouse, Ph.D., R.N., F.A.A.N.

Wayne State University, Detroit, MI

Research on adjustment to breast cancer has moved from examining adjustment at one point in time to examining adjustment at multiple time points over the course of illness. This shift in focus has enabled investigators and clinicans to develop a broader understanding of the process of adjustment and to identify critical time points for intervention. The research by Hoskins and colleagues extends the existing research base and provides valuable information about the relationship between social support and adjustment during the first year following diagnosis.

It is commendable that the investigators conducted this study with a large sample of women ($N = 128$) and their husbands (husband data are reported in another article), used six assessment times that started 7-10 days postdiagnosis and continued until 1 year postsurgery, and used established instruments to measure multiple study variables. Based on a review of literature, they specified the relationships that they expected to find among the study variables and tested most of these relationships.

There are a number of challenges that face investigators conducting longitudinal studies on adjustment to breast cancer. One challenge is determining how to measure "adjustment." Although most investigators agree that it is a multidimensional construct that includes physical and emotional components, it has been measured in many different ways across studies, making it difficult to compare findings (See Irvine, Brown, Crooks, Roberts, & Brown, 1991 for a review). In this study, the investigators took a multidimensional approach and measured emotional adjustment, physical adjustment, and health status. Social adjustment was not measured as an outcome variable but was assessed as a predictor variable called functional status. They also used multiple indicators of each outcome variable which was a strength.

Another interesting way of dealing with the data would be to create indexes for each outcome variable from the multiple indicators (e.g., an emotional adjustment index from the three indicators) rather than conduct separate analyses for each indicator across the six data points.

A second challenge investigators face is controlling for the effects of initial adjustment on subsequent measures of adjustment. Stanton and Snider (1993) found that women's emotional distress prior to breast biopsy was significantly related to their adjustment following biopsy. Similarly, Dean (1987) found that preoperative distress was a significant predictor of women's adjustment 3 months following mastectomy. In this study, adjustment was measured at six points in time, and it would be helpful to know the extent to which initial emotional adjustment was correlated with later emotional adjustment.

A third challenge investigators face is determining how to measure "patterns" of adjustment. In this study the investigators reported a series of correlations between social support and emotional adjustment and physical adjustment over the six assessment times. This information was helpful and illustrated the ongoing relationship between support and emotional adjustment. Further analysis of this rich dataset using Repeated Measures Analysis of Variance would provide additional information about women's patterns of adjustment. Were there significant changes in women's levels of emotional adjustment or physical adjustment during the first year following diagnosis? Was there a decrease in women's psychological distress over time as reported by some investigators (Goldberg et al., 1992) or was there a sustained pattern of distress as reported by others (Northouse, 1989)? At which assessment time did women experience the greatest number of emotional symptoms or physical symptoms? Answers to questions such as these would further clarify the process of adjustment and identify key points for intervention.

There were a number of important findings reported in this study that have implications for clinical practice. First, the findings underscore the importance of support from the woman's marital partner. A number of investigators have examined the relationship between *amount* of support (globally defined) and adjustment, but they seldom have identified who is the *source* of the support. Results of this study point to the key role that spouses play during the first year following diagnosis. The results also indicate that it is important to assess initial levels of marital support because they are significantly related to women's adjustment 1 year later.

It is important to note, however, that spouses often do not feel prepared for this primary support role (Sabo, Brown, & Smith, 1986). They often feel overwhelmed by the demands of the illness and uncertain about how to help their wives (Zahlis & Shands, 1991). Furthermore, they have little contact with health professionals (Northouse, 1988) and hence little opportunity to receive information and support from professionals. Health professionals need to investigate the informational and support needs of spouses and find ways to strengthen their alliances with them. This will help facilitate spouses' adjustment to their wives' illness and provide spouses with the resources that they need to support their wives.

Other close interpersonal friends and extended family members were also important sources of support for women in this study. Similar to marital support, support from these two sources early in the course of illness (7-10 days) was significantly related to women's adjustment at 1 year. Of these two sources of support, stronger and more consistent relationships were found between women's adjustment and their support from close interpersonal relationships rather than from extended family. The weaker relationships associated with extended family support are probably related to the fact that it was measured with a 4-item subscale of the PAIS (with low internal consistency) that focused primarily on "contact" with extended family members rather than perceived support. Nevertheless, the findings indicate that other sources of support, in addition to marital support, are related to women's emotional adjustment over time.

Another important finding reported in this study was related to women's perceived health status. Women who reported greater satisfaction with the attitude of health care professionals and the information that they received from them reported fewer health problems. Few studies have examined the behavior of health professionals and its relationship to client outcomes, but the findings of this study suggest that this is an area that warrants continued study. Further analyses need to take into account the effect of demographic and medical variables on women's satisfaction with health care and on the number of health problems they report over time. For example, do younger women report greater or lesser satisfaction with health care? Does the type of adjuvant treatment women receive affect their satisfaction with health care or the type of problems they report over time? Medical history variables need to be considered in conjunction with other psychosocial factors to understand the complexity of factors that affect women's perception of their health.

Finally, this longitudinal study provided important information about predictors evident early in the course of illness that relate to adjustment at 6 months and 1 year. As reported by Hoskins and colleagues women who perceived more support, greater satisfaction with their health care, and fewer role problems early in the course of illness, had better adjustment at 6 months and 1 year. This information is very valuable. It directs professionals to assess women's support resources, satisfaction with care, and functional status early in the course of illness, and to intervene when problems are evident. More studies are needed that identify other early predictors of long-term adjustment to breast cancer. From a series of studies, we will be able identify a profile of factors that place women and their partners at risk of poorer adjustment over time. This valuable information cannot be obtained from cross-sectional studies. More longitudinal studies are needed that provide information on patterns and predictors of adjustment that can be used to direct clinical practice.

REFERENCES

Dean, C. (1987). Psychiatric morbidity following mastectomy: Preoperative predictors and types of illness. *Journal of Psychosomatic Research, 31*, 385-392.

Goldberg, J.A., Scott, R.N., Davidson, P.M., Murray, G.D., Stallard, S., George, W.D., & Maguire, G.P. (1992). Psychological morbidity in the first year after breast surgery. *European Journal of Surgical Oncology, 18*, 327-331.

Irvine, D., Brown, B., Crooks, D., Roberts, J., & Browne, G. (1991). Psychosocial adjustment in women with breast cancer. *Cancer, 67*, 1097-1117.

Northouse, L.L.(1988). Social support in patients' and husbands' adjustment to breast cancer. *Nursing Research, 37*, 91-95.

Northouse, L.L. (1989). A longitudinal study of the adjustment of patients and husbands to breast cancer. *Oncology Nursing Forum, 16*, 511-516.

Sabo, D., Brown, J., & Smith, C. (1986). The male role and mastectomy: Support groups and men's adjustment. *Journal of Psychosocial Oncology, 4*, 19-31.

Stanton, A. L., & Snider, P.R. (1993). Coping with a breast cancer diagnosis: A prospective study. *Health Psychology, 12*, 16-23.

Zahlis, E.H., & Shands, M.E. (1991). Breast cancer: Demands of illness on the patients' partner. *Journal of Psychosocial Oncology, 9*, 75-93.

Offprints. Requests for offprints should be directed to Laurel Northouse, Ph.D., R.N., F.A.A.N., College of Nursing, Wayne State University, 5557 Cass Avenue, Detroit, MI 48202.

Appendix D

Testing Hypotheses with an Exemplar Study: Statistical Significance, Error, Directionality, and Power

From: Waltz, C., & Bausell, R. B. (1981). *Nursing research: Design, statistics and computer analysis* (pp. 19–29). Philadelphia: F. A. Davis.

Ex. "Consider two groups of subjects, one having received preoperative instruction regarding what they could expect from their surgical experience, the other having received only the usual hospital routine" (p. 19).

"If these groups were to be compared with respect to the amount of postoperative medication they required, then all that would seemingly be necessary to test the null hypothesis would be to count up the number of times patients in each group requested medication and see if one group requested more than the other. Theoretically, it would seem that if the group that received the preoperative instruction requested exactly the same amount of medication as the group that did not receive instruction, there would be no relationship between preoperative instruction and medication requests" (pp. 19–20).

"Under such conditions, the null hypothesis would be considered to be probably true (that is, H_0 = 'Patients receiving preoperative instruction do not differ from patients not receiving preoperative instruction with respect to the amount of medication requested following surgery')."

"With this particular outcome, such a conclusion would be difficult to refute. What, however, if the experimental group (that is, those subjects receiving preoperative instruction) had requested medication a total of 78 times and the control group's requests had totaled 79? Would the researcher be justified in arguing that the null hypothesis was probably false and that a relationship did indeed exist between the variables? Would a hospital administrator be justified in authorizing preoperative instruction for all patients on the basis of this minute difference between groups?"

"The probability is that after a little thought a reasonable administrator would conclude that the difference was too small to be sure that preoperative instruction had any real effect upon requests for medication. Such a decision would be correct because, in research dealing with different groups of people under different conditions, results are almost never identical across groups, people, and time. Given two or more groups, in fact, it is far more likely that in the final analysis these groups will differ to some degree than it is that they will not differ at all. Given this state of affairs, therefore, it should be obvious that some objective criterion should be available to ascertain whether or not a hypothesized relationship should be accepted as 'real' or rejected as not real. Such a criterion does exist. It is called statistical significance and it is basic to all hypothesis testing" (p. 20).

I.   CONCEPT OF STATISTICAL SIGNIFICANCE

    A.   "The substitution of a statistical value for an observed relationship or difference"
    B.   "The comparison of the statistical value to a distribution of other statistical values to determine how likely such a value (and hence the relationship it represents) would be to occur by chance alone

        1.   If the odds are on the side of the observed relationship not occurring by chance alone, then the H_0 is considered probably false (and H_1 probably true)."
        2.   "If the odds seem to favor the relationship occurring by chance, then the H_0 is accepted as probably true" (p. 20).

    Ex.   "Suppose the results in the following table had occurred when conducting the above-mentioned study contrasting a group of patients receiving preoperative instruction with a group receiving no instruction with respect to requests for medication following surgery" (p. 20).

"Patients receiving preoperative instruction appeared to request pain medications less frequently than control patients: the former registering 11 requests as opposed to 25 for the latter. The question becomes, since it is unlikely that the two groups would have registered identical medication requests regardless of the experimental treatment (instruction), is the difference actually observed (that is, $25 - 11 = 14$) likely to have occurred by chance alone? If the answer is no, then the researcher can conclude that the observed difference (14) was due to the fact that one group received preoperative instruction and the other did not (if the study was conducted carefully) and that H_0 could be rejected as probably false. If the answer

TABLE D.1 **Hypothetical Postoperative Medication Requests of Patients Who Received and Patients Who Did Not Receive Preoperative Instruction (p. 21)**

	E (instruction)		C (no instruction)	
Patient	Number of requests		Patient	Number of requests
#1	3		#5	4
#2	2		#6	6
#3	1		#7	8
#4	5		#8	7
Total	11		Total	25

is yes, then the researcher would conclude that the instruction had no measurable effect and that H_0 was probably correct" (pp. 20–21).

"The actual decision of whether or not H_0 should be considered probably true or probably false is easy to make. Conceptually, the process consists of two steps: (1) determining the level of error that can be tolerated in reaching the decision, and (2) determining how likely the actual results obtained were to have occurred by chance alone" (p. 21).

II.   LEVEL OF ERROR

A.   In behavioral research, the maximum tolerable error for considering the H_0 probably false is 5% (researchers are willing to be wrong 5 times out of 100 when rejecting the H_0)

1.   called the "alpha level" or "level of significance"

Probability of obtained results occurring by chance

A.   "Determine how likely the actual results obtained were to have occurred by chance alone

1.   choose an appropriate statistic to represent the relationship
2.   compute the statistic (= translating the relationship in such a way that it can be represented by the numerical value of the statistic)
3.   compare the statistic to its particular distribution to see how likely it (and hence the relationship it represents) was to occur by chance alone."

Ex.   "Given the eight medication requests observed in the study (e.g., 3, 2, 1, 5, 4, 6, 8, and 7), what is the probability that a difference as large as 14 (25 − 11) would occur by chance alone?" (p. 22).

TABLE D.2 Examples of Possible Combinations for the Two Groups of Four Numbers

(1)		(2)		(3)		(4)		(5)		(6)	
E	C	E	C	E	C	E	C	E	C	E	C
1	5	1	4	1	2	1	2	2	1	5	1
2	6	2	6	3	4	3	4	3	4	6	2
3	7	3	7	6	5	6	5	6	5	7	3
4	8	5	8	7	8	8	7	7	8	8	4
10	26	11	25	17	19	18	18	18	18	26	10
	16		14		2		0		0		16

TABLE D.3 Frequency Distribution of Differences Between the Two Groups (p. 24)

Differences between E and C totals	Total number of unique combinations that can produce these differences
16	2
14	2
12	4
10	6
8	10
6	10
4	14
2	14
0	8
	70

"The total number of combinations of two groups of four numbers each can easily be calculated mathematically (by computer for large amounts of data). Starting with the eight numbers listed in the previous table, it is possible to construct 70 different combinations, of which having the numbers 3, 2, 1, and 5 in the experimental group and 4, 6, 8, and 7 in the control is only one (a few of these combinations are in the table below)."

"The researcher could then compute differences between these 70 unique combinations of four numbers and construct a frequency distribution of the differences between the two groups (see table below). Note that although there are 70 different combinations of four numbers possible, there are not 70 unique differences between groups" (p. 23).

"This frequency distribution represents all the possible chance differences that could occur between the two groups of four numbers and the possible ways in which each difference can occur. Once constructed, all the researcher need do to determine how likely the observed difference of 14 was to occur by chance alone is to determine how many ways a difference of 14 or greater could occur and divide that figure by the total number of unique combinations of two groups of four numbers each.

"Referring to the distribution, it is found that there are two ways by which the difference of 14 could have occurred by chance and two ways by which an even greater difference

APPENDIX D

(16) could have occurred. This means that a difference as great as 14 could have occurred by chance a total of 4 times out of 70; thus the probability that the observed 14 did occur by chance alone is 4 divided by 70 or 0.057. If the level of significance or alpha level of this study had been set at 0.05, which is likely, then the null hypothesis could not be rejected because the researcher would be wrong 5.7 out of 100 times rather than the permissible 5 out of 100" (p. 24).

III. DIRECTIONALITY

"In the above study, the researcher tested the following H_1: 'Patients receiving preoperative instruction differ significantly from patients not receiving preoperative instruction with respect to number of postoperative medication requests.' Given this non-directional hypothesis, a difference of 14 favoring the control group would receive the same treatment as the observed difference of 14 favoring the experimental group. A very different situation would exist, however, if the researcher had posited a direction to the relationship" (pp. 24–25).

Ex. "Suppose the following H_0 had been tested: 'Patients receiving preoperative instruction register significantly fewer postoperative medication requests than patients not receiving preoperative instruction' " (p. 25).

"In this situation, unlike the previous one, a difference of 14 favoring the control group would not receive the same treatment as the observed difference of 14 favoring the experimental group. The reason for this should be clear. H_1 posited a significant (that is, an alpha of 0.05 or less) difference between the groups *favoring* the experimental group; hence any difference favoring the control group would be considered supportive of H_0, not H_1. In other words, no matter how great a difference observed in favor of the control group, H_1 would be automatically rejected as probably false."

"Given the directional H_1 positing a difference favoring the experimental group therefore, a question arises concerning how to redefine differences occurring by chance and consequently how to determine the probability of a difference as large as 14 *favoring the experimental* group occurring by chance."

"The above table can no longer be used because no distinctions were made between the direction of the difference between the experimental and control groups. Referring to that distribution indicates, for example, that from the total 70 unique combinations of groups of four numbers, two could be expected to produce differences as large as 16 and two produce differences as large as 14. In actuality, only one combination was capable of producing a difference of 16 favoring the experimental group (that is, E = 1, 2, 3, and 4; C = 5, 6, 7, and 8), the other difference of 16 favored the control group (that is, E = 5, 6, 7, and 8; C = 1, 2, 3, and 4) as indicated in the third table above. The same held for differences of 14; only one unique combination of the 70 possible favored the experimental group; the other consisted of a mirror image favoring the control group.

"To ascertain the probability of a 14 favoring E when such a direction had been hypothesized a priori, therefore, the researcher would count only the single difference of 16 and the single difference of 14 favoring the experimental group, and would ignore the 16 and 14 differences favoring the control group. Thus, instead of dividing 4 (two differences of 16 and two of 14) by 70, the researcher would divide 2 by 70 and obtain 0.0285 instead of 0.057, thereby rejecting H_0 as probably false and accepting H_1 as probably true.

"In other words, if everything else is equal, the same difference is half as likely to occur by chance in a directional hypothesis as in a nondirectional one *if that difference occurs in the proper direction*" (p. 25).

Summary:

1. The number of requests for each member of the E group and for each member of the C group are determined.
2. All possible combinations of numbers of requests by E subjects with numbers of requests by C subjects are computed.
3. The number of requests for the E group and for the C group are totaled for each combination.
4. The difference is calculated for each combination.
5. A frequency distribution of the differences represents all the possible chance differences that could occur and the possible ways in which each difference can occur.

   > *Assumption*: In a nondirectional hypothesis, the direction is not considered. E = 10; C = 14; difference = −4. (Those who have preop teaching will make fewer requests.) Also included, however, is E = 14; C = 10; difference = +4.

6. The researcher now can determine how likely the observed difference between the E group and C group in *their* study could occur by chance alone.

   > *Procedure*: Divide the calculated difference by the total number of unique combinations. If the value is less than the set alpha, or significance level, H_0 can be rejected. (The researcher has been wrong less than 5 times out of 100 if *p* is set at .05 and the above value is less).

7. In the case of a directional hypothesis, a difference favoring the C group does not receive the same treatment as a difference favoring the E group. The researcher in this case divides the calculated difference favoring the E group only by the total number of unique combinations.

IV. POWER

"There are only two possible decisions that can be made when testing a null hypothesis: the researcher can reject it as probably false or accept it as probably true. In each case, the decision can either be right or wrong, although the researcher can never be sure which. It is possible, however, to estimate how likely the decision to reject H_0 was to be incorrect by computing the significance level of the relationship, sometimes called the probability of Type I error, which of course implies the existence of a Type II error as well.

"Type II error occurs only when the researcher *fails* to reject H_0. In this case Type I error is completely irrelevant, but obviously error could be present just as easily in failing to find a significant relationship as in finding one. Just as obviously, the researcher will never know for sure whether the decision to accept H_0 as probably true is right or wrong, but again the likelihood of making such an error can be estimated although the process is more complex.

"At first glance, these two sources of error may appear to be independent of one another since only one genre need be considered for any one study (Type I error is irrelevant when failing to reject H_0; Type II irrelevant when succeeding in rejecting H_0). The two concepts are very closely related. The reason for this is probably best illustrated through the concept of power and its relationship to statistical significance.

"Power is defined as the probability of rejecting the null hypothesis when it should be rejected (that is, when in 'reality' it is false) and is really nothing more than 1 minus Type II error. Since statistical significance determines whether or not the null hypothesis is rejected, the same parameters that influence statistical significance also influence power (and hence Type II error). Power, then, like statistical significance, is a function of the alpha set by the researcher prior to the study (the more stringent the alpha, the lower the power), the homogeneity of the subjects (the more homogeneous the criterion scores within groups, the greater the power), the difference between the groups with respect to the dependent variable (the greater the difference between groups, the greater the power), and the relative size of the sample (the more subjects participating in a study, the greater the power)" (p. 27).

Index

Springer Publishing Company

From the Springer Series on The Teaching of Nursing...

Developing An Online Course
Best Practices for Nurse Educators

Carol A. O'Neil, PhD, RN
Cheryl A. Fisher, MSN, RN
Susan K. Newbold, MSN, RNBC, FAAN

This book takes educators through the necessary steps to transform a traditional course into an online or partially online course —which may be part of a traditional nursing education program, a continuing education course, or a certification program. The authors address questions such as: How can learning theories be applied online? What does "class participation" mean online? What are options for clinical lab experiences? What sort of technical support will I need?

Readers will find invaluable a decision tree outlining each step in the process as well as a sample course syllabus showing the day-by-day structure of an online course.

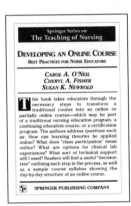

Contents:

- Introduction to Web-Based Teaching and Learning
- Theories of Learning and the Online Environment
- Developing the Infrastructure for Online Learning: Student, Faculty, and Technical Support
- Technologies and Competencies Needed for Online Learning
- Reconceptualizing the Online Course
- Designing the Online Learning Environment
- Course Management Methods
- Interacting and Communicating Online
- Assessment and Evaluation of Online Learning

2004   184pp   0-8261-2546-8   hard

11 West 42nd Street, New York, NY 10036-8002 • Fax: 212-941-7842
Order Toll-Free: 877-687-7476 • Order On-line: www.springerpub.com

Springer Publishing Company

From the Springer Series on The Teaching of Nursing…

Teaching Nursing in an Associate Degree Program

Rita G. Mertig, MS, RNC, CNS

"Content is presented in a straightforward manner…covers the most significant topics central to entry-level nursing education."

—From the Foreword by **Joyce Fitzpatrick**, PhD, RN, FAAN

This practical "how to" book for teaching nursing in an associate degree program is for new and not-so-new faculty. Advice gleaned from the author's many years of teaching is presented in a friendly and easy-to-read format, designed to quickly help new faculty get a positive sense of direction.

The special issues of AD nursing students—many have full-time jobs, families, and are more mature than the "traditional" college student—are given full consideration. Strategies discussed include: What to do during the first class • Motivating students • Helping the student in crisis • Helping students with poor reading, study, and academic skills • Helping students with time management

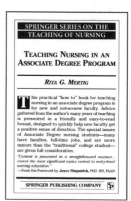

Contents:

2003   128pp   0-8261-2004-0   hard

11 West 42nd Street, New York, NY 10036-8002 • **Fax: 212-941-7842**
Order Toll-Free: 877-687-7476 • **Order On-line: www.springerpub.com**